Transcranial Magnetic Stimulation

Clinical Applications for Psychiatric Practice

Second Edition

T0295346

Transcranial Magnetic Stimulation

Clinical Applications for Psychiatric Practice

Second Edition

Edited by

Richard A. Bermudes, M.D.
Karl I. Lanocha, M.D.
Philip G. Janicak, M.D.

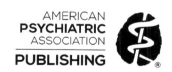

AMERICAN
PSYCHIATRIC
ASSOCIATION
PUBLISHING

If you wish to buy 50 or more copies of the same title, please go to www.appi.org/specialdiscounts for more information.

American Psychiatric Association Publishing
800 Maine Avenue SW, Suite 900
Washington, DC 20024-2812
www.appi.org

Library of Congress Cataloging-in-Publication Data
Names: Bermudes, Richard A., 1967- editor. | Lanocha, Karl I., editor. | Janicak, Philip G., editor. | American Psychiatric Association Publishing, issuing body.
Title: Transcranial magnetic stimulation : clinical applications for psychiatric practice / edited by Richard A. Bermudes, Karl I. Lanocha, Philip G. Janicak.
Other titles: Transcranial magnetic stimulation (Bermudes)
Description: Second edition. | Washington, D.C. : American Psychiatric Association Publishing, [2025] | Includes bibliographical references and index.
Identifiers: LCCN 2024029349 (print) | LCCN 2024029350 (ebook) | ISBN 9798894550657 (paperback ; alk. paper) | ISBN 9798894550664 (ebook)
Subjects: MESH: Transcranial Magnetic Stimulation | Depressive Disorder, Major--therapy
Classification: LCC RC386.2 (print) | LCC RC386.2 (ebook) | NLM WM 171.5 | DDC 616.89/12--dc23/eng/20240715
LC record available at https://lccn.loc.gov/2024029349
LC ebook record available at https://lccn.loc.gov/2024029350

British Library Cataloguing in Publication Data
A CIP record is available from the British Library.

Contents

Contributors vii

Introduction xi
Richard A. Bermudes, M.D., Karl I. Lanocha, M.D., and
Philip G. Janicak, M.D.

In Memoriam: Karl I. Lanocha, M.D. xv

1   Basic Principles of Transcranial Magnetic Stimulation . . . 1
Karl I. Lanocha, M.D., Richard A. Bermudes, M.D., and
Philip G. Janicak, M.D.

2   Transcranial Magnetic Stimulation Therapy for
    Major Depression 25
Karl I. Lanocha, M.D., Richard A. Bermudes, M.D., and
Philip G. Janicak, M.D.

3   Integrating Pharmacotherapy and Psychotherapy
    With Transcranial Magnetic Stimulation for
    Major Depressive Disorder. 63
Mehmet E. Dokucu, M.D., Ph.D., Richard A. Bermudes, M.D.,
and Philip G. Janicak, M.D.

4   Transcranial Magnetic Stimulation for the
    Treatment of Other Mood Disorders 91
Juan F. Garzon, M.D., Scott T. Aaronson, M.D., and
Paul E. Croarkin, D.O., M.S.

5 Risk Management Issues in Transcranial Magnetic Stimulation for Treatment of Major Depression 117
Philip G. Janicak, M.D., and Richard A. Bermudes, M.D.

6 Transcranial Magnetic Stimulation for OCD 135
Richard A. Bermudes, M.D., and Philip G. Janicak, M.D.

7 Transcranial Magnetic Stimulation for Disorders Other Than Depression 163
Karl I. Lanocha, M.D., Richard A. Bermudes, M.D., and Philip G. Janicak, M.D.

8 Transcranial Magnetic Stimulation and Other Neuromodulation Therapies 183
Karl I. Lanocha, M.D., Richard A. Bermudes, M.D., and Philip G. Janicak, M.D.

9 Current FDA-Cleared Transcranial Magnetic Stimulation Systems 201
Ian A. Cook, M.D., and Richard A. Bermudes, M.D.

10 Transcranial Magnetic Stimulation: Recent and Future Innovations 235
Ian A. Cook, M.D., Richard A. Bermudes, M.D., and Philip G. Janicak, M.D.

11 Clinical Applications and Patient Selection: Who Should Be Referred for Transcranial Magnetic Stimulation Therapy? 259
Karl I. Lanocha, M.D., Richard A. Bermudes, M.D., and Philip G. Janicak, M.D.

12 Important Practice Management Tips for Transcranial Magnetic Stimulation Clinicians 277
Richard A. Bermudes, M.D.

Appendix: Transcranial Magnetic Stimulation Training Courses 309
Richard A. Bermudes, M.D.

Index 315

Contributors

Scott T. Aaronson, M.D.

Chief Science Officer, Institute for Advanced Diagnostics and Therapeutics, and Director of Clinical Research, Sheppard Pratt Health System, Baltimore, Maryland; Adjunct Professor of Psychiatry, University of Maryland School of Medicine, Baltimore, Maryland

Richard A. Bermudes, M.D.

President, Empathy MindCare, Zephyr Cove, Nevada; Associate Physician, Department of Psychiatry and Behavioral Sciences, University of California, Davis, Sacramento, California

Ian A. Cook, M.D.

Director, CEO, and Founder, Los Angeles TMS Institute; Professor Emeritus of Psychiatry and of Bioengineering, University of California, Los Angeles, California

Paul E. Croarkin, D.O., M.S.

Professor of Pediatrics, Pharmacology, and Psychiatry and Ervin A. and Margaret C. Mueller Director, Mayo Clinic Children's Research Center, Mayo Clinic, Rochester, Minnesota

Mehmet E. Dokucu, M.D., Ph.D.

Director of Mood Disorders and Interventional Psychiatry, Associate Professor of Psychiatry, Dartmouth Geisel School of Medicine, Hanover, New Hampshire

Juan F. Garzon, M.D.
Research Fellow, Department of Psychiatry and Psychology, Mayo Clinic, Rochester, Minnesota

Philip G. Janicak, M.D.
Adjunct Professor and Consultant to the Neuromodulation Center, Department of Psychiatry and Behavioral Sciences, Northwestern University Feinberg School of Medicine, Chicago, Illinois

Karl I. Lanocha, M.D.[†]
Director of Education, Mindful Health Solutions, San Francisco, California

Disclosure of Competing Interests

The following contributors to this book have indicated a financial interest in or other affiliation with a commercial supporter, a manufacturer of a commercial product, a provider of a commercial service, a nongovernmental organization, and/or a government agency, as listed below:

Scott T. Aaronson, M.D., served as a paid consultant to Neuronetics, LivaNova, Genomind, and Sage Therapeutics. Dr. Aaronson has received research support from Compass Pathways.

Richard A. Bermudes, M.D., has received equity, 1099, and affiliations from Mindful Health Solutions, American Psychiatric Association Publishing Inc., and Clinical TMS Society; common shares and performance value units from TMS HP, LLC (Norwest Venture Partners); and W-2 from Mindful Health Solutions.

Ian A. Cook, M.D., has received National Institutes of Health grants to Stanford University and to University of Southern California (Data and Safety Monitoring Board, consultant). He served as the site primary investigator for Magnus Medical. He has patents assigned to NeuroSigma and HeartCloud. Dr. Cook is a shareholder at Los Angeles TMS Institute, HeartCloud, and NeuroSigma. He holds volunteer positions on the Board of Directors, Clinical TMS Society, and Board of Directors and Vice President, Foundation for the Advancement of Clinical TMS. Dr. Cook is employed by Los Angeles TMS Institute (private practice) and was previously Chief Medical Officer & Senior Vice President of NeuroSigma, Inc., and CEO and Co-Founder of HeartCloud, Inc.

[†]Deceased.

Paul E. Croarkin, D.O., M.S., has received research support from the National Institutes of Health (NIH), the National Science Foundation (NSF), the Brain and Behavior Research Foundation, the Mayo Clinic Foundation, and Pfizer, Inc. He has received equipment support from Neuronetics, Inc., and MagVenture, Inc. He received grant-in-kind supplies and genotyping from Assurex Health, Inc., for an investigator-initiated study. He served as the primary investigator for a multicenter study funded by Neuronetics, Inc. and a site primary investigator for a study funded by NeoSync, Inc. Dr. Croarkin served as a paid consultant for Engrail Therapeutics, Sunovion, Procter & Gamble Company, Meta Platforms, Inc., and Myriad Neuroscience. Dr. Croarkin is employed by Mayo Clinic.

Mehmet E. Dokucu, M.D., Ph.D., has received honoraria and travel expenses for the Clinical TMS Society Pulses Training Course.

Philip G. Janicak, M.D., has received support from TMS Solutions, Neuronetics, and American Psychiatric Association Publishing Inc.

The following contributors have indicated that they have no financial interests or other affiliations that represent or could appear to represent a competing interest with their contributions to this book during the year preceding manuscript submission:

Juan F. Garzon, M.D.
Karl I. Lanocha, M.D.

Introduction

Richard A. Bermudes, M.D.
Karl I. Lanocha, M.D.
Philip G. Janicak, M.D.

Psychiatric disorders represent a significant and growing societal problem (GBD 2019 Mental Disorders Collaborators 2022). In addition to being a leading cause of disability worldwide, many of these disorders increase the risk for medical conditions such as coronary artery disease and diabetes, two leading causes of morbidity and mortality (Druss et al. 2011; Osborn et al. 2008). Although many patients' symptoms are effectively treated with pharmacotherapy, psychotherapy, or a combination, up to 30% of patients with mood and anxiety conditions do not respond to these standard treatments (Bystritsky 2006; Rush et al. 2006).

In October 2008, the first transcranial magnetic stimulation (TMS) system was cleared by the FDA to treat major depressive disorder in adult patients whose symptoms had not responded to one antidepressant medication. This marked the beginning of psychiatry's most important treatment development in the past two decades.

Since the first edition of this book, the field of TMS has seen remarkable growth, transitioning from a period of promising research to the development of numerous medical devices that have received FDA clearance for OCD, anxiety comorbid with major depressive disorder, and smoking cessation.

Furthermore, insurance coverage for TMS has expanded, with many insurance companies covering TMS after one to two treatment failures. This diversification highlights the technology's potential and the strides being made to incorporate noninvasive therapeutic neuromodulation into mental health treatment.

Despite the growing availability of this innovative option, many practitioners still need to determine how to use TMS best. This lack of clarity is partly because most psychiatric residency programs do not offer any TMS curriculum or clinical training, and continuing education conferences are limited.

This book provides mental health practitioners with a practical reference for managing patients who are candidates for TMS. In this context, we discuss the integration of TMS with psychotherapy, pharmacotherapy, and other forms of neuromodulation; the identification of appropriate patients for referral to a TMS clinician; the coordination of care by the primary treatment team and TMS service to ensure the best outcomes during the acute, continuation, and maintenance treatment phases of depression; and the evolving nature of TMS research, such as the ongoing development of TMS and related technologies. The appendix lists various options for advanced TMS training, both theoretical and hands-on, sponsored by specialty societies and medical centers.

The chapter authors are clinician-researchers with extensive knowledge of TMS's clinical applications and other forms of neuromodulation. The discussion in Chapter 1, "Basic Principles of Transcranial Magnetic Stimulation," covers the development of TMS, an overview of parameters, and the mechanism of action. The following chapters review the literature for a particular topic and provide one or more clinical vignettes highlighting how TMS is integrated into patient care. Although the TMS literature has grown exponentially in the past two decades, clinicians must still manage patients whose histories may differ from those of study populations. Therefore, each chapter lists key points that summarize the optimal clinical application of TMS for the general mental health provider. In summary, this work provides an update on the current clinical role of TMS and a road map to its potential future.

References

Bystritsky A: Treatment-resistant anxiety disorders. Mol Psychiatry 11(9):805–814, 2006 16847460

Druss BG, Zhao L, Von Esenwein S, et al: Understanding excess mortality in persons with mental illness: 17-year follow up of a nationally representative US survey. Med Care 49(6):599–604, 2011 21577183

GBD 2019 Mental Disorders Collaborators: Global, regional, and national burden of 12 mental disorders in 204 countries and territories, 1990–2019: a systematic analysis for the Global Burden of Disease Study 2019. Lancet Psychiatry 9(2):137–150, 2022 35026139

Osborn DP, Wright CA, Levy G, et al: Relative risk of diabetes, dyslipidaemia, hypertension and the metabolic syndrome in people with severe mental illnesses: systematic review and metaanalysis. BMC Psychiatry 8:84, 2008 18817565

Rush AJ, Trivedi MH, Wisniewski SR, et al: Acute and longer-term outcomes in depressed outpatients requiring one or several treatment steps: a STAR*D report. Am J Psychiatry 163(11):1905–1917, 2006 17074942

In Memoriam: Karl I. Lanocha, M.D.

It is with heavy hearts that we remember and honor the remarkable life and contributions of Karl I. Lanocha, M.D., a true pioneer in transcranial magnetic stimulation (TMS) therapy. Dr. Lanocha's legacy continues to resonate within our hearts and minds, and his effect on the broader psychiatric community is immeasurable.

Dr. Lanocha was one of the earliest adopters of TMS in clinical practice, paving the way for countless others in the field. His pioneering spirit led him to establish the first TMS therapy clinic at Concord Hospital, New Hampshire, shortly after the FDA cleared the first device for clinical use in the United States in 2008.

Beyond his clinical practice, Dr. Lanocha was a devoted educator and advocate for TMS therapy. His eloquent and inspiring talks on the prescription of TMS therapy were transformative for many clinicians, altering the course of their careers. He tirelessly trained hundreds of physicians, ensuring that TMS therapy reached thousands of patients.

Dr. Lanocha played a pivotal role in the inception of the Clinical TMS Society, serving as a founding member of its board of directors. His commitment to advancing the field through translational psychiatry and therapeutic neuromodulation was unwavering. In this context, Dr. Lanocha's clinical expertise spanned TMS therapy, psychotherapy, pharmacotherapy, electroconvulsive therapy, and novel treatments such as ketamine and esketamine.

In memory of Dr. Lanocha, we recognize his exceptional contributions to TMS therapy, the Clinical TMS Society, and this book's editions. His legacy serves as an inspiration to those who follow in his footsteps. We are profoundly grateful for his remarkable life, the opportunity to work closely with him, and his enduring effect on clinical psychiatry.

Basic Principles of Transcranial Magnetic Stimulation

Karl I. Lanocha, M.D.
Richard A. Bermudes, M.D.
Philip G. Janicak, M.D.

Transcranial magnetic stimulation (TMS) is a noninvasive method of stimulating the human brain. The stimulation is produced with a brief, high-intensity, pulsed magnetic field generated by an electrical current passing through a coil of wire, known as the *magnetic coil*. In turn, the magnetic field induces an electrical field capable of depolarizing a localized brain area beneath the coil. TMS can modulate brain activity without surgery or anesthesia. Although it is widely used in neuroscience research, it also has several diagnostic and therapeutic applications.

1

Depression was the first FDA-cleared therapeutic application for TMS and remains an important breakthrough for several reasons:

- TMS is effective for patients who do not respond to conventional medication and/or psychotherapy.
- Unlike electroconvulsive therapy (ECT), TMS is an office-based procedure that does not induce a seizure and requires no anesthesia or sedation.
- Unlike ECT, TMS causes no cognitive adverse effects.
- Unlike medication, TMS causes no systemic adverse effects, such as weight gain or sexual dysfunction.
- Unlike medication treatment, which is prone to patient error and nonadherence, TMS is an observed procedure during which the clinician can ensure proper administration.

Although most studies regarding its clinical application currently focus on treating depression, it is important to understand at the outset that TMS is not an antidepressant per se. Instead, TMS is better understood as a circuit or network modulator. The clinical effects of TMS depend on which brain circuit or network is stimulated and how that stimulation is applied.

Since the initial FDA device clearance, many TMS systems have become available. They differ in engineering and design elements, including the electromagnetic coil configuration, leading to a growing number of clinical applications. These applications include OCD, nicotine dependence (smoking cessation), and migraine headaches. Other potential indications include schizophrenia, bipolar disorder, chronic pain, and cognitive impairment.

In this chapter, we provide an overview of TMS. It begins with a history of its development, followed by an explanation of basic principles and an overview of how different stimulation parameters affect brain function. We conclude with a discussion of TMS's putative mechanisms of action in treating depression.

Historical Development of TMS

TMS is a form of brain electrical stimulation without the use of electrodes. It is a clinical application of Faraday's law of induction, whose fundamental principles have been understood for almost two centuries (Faraday 1831/1965). Electricity and magnetism are two aspects of the same phenomenon. Every electrical current creates a magnetic field in the surrounding space, whereas a time-varying or moving magnetic field can induce an electrical current in a nearby conductor. In the case of TMS, the electrical conductor is the human nervous system (Figure 1–1).

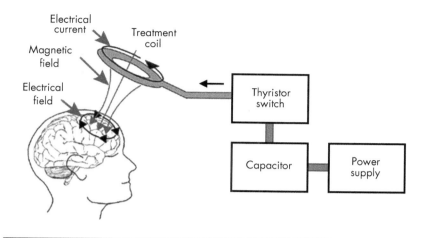

Figure 1–1. Flow of electrical current in nearby neural tissue caused by a moving magnetic field.

Although not depicted in this illustration, the transcranial magnetic stimulation coil must be in direct contact with the patient's scalp to produce an electrical field strong enough to cause depolarization.

Soon after Faraday's discovery and the recognition that living tissues are conductive, studies began to test the effects of changing magnetic fields on excitable tissues. The first serious investigations of magnetic stimulation of human nervous tissue began in the late nineteenth and early twentieth centuries. In 1896, French physician and physicist Jacques-Arsène d'Arsonval induced phosphenes (perceived flashes of light without photic stimulation) in human subjects standing inside a 2-meter-high solenoid made of thick copper wire. This was likely the first demonstration that a magnetic field could alter human brain function noninvasively (Theodore 2002). Magnetically induced phosphenes were a subject of considerable interest when Nikola Tesla attempted to develop an alternating current for commercial use. In 1910, British engineer Sylvanus P. Thompson demonstrated phosphene induction by magnetic stimulation of the occipital cortex (Thompson 1910). Although electromagnetism was occasionally used in basic neuroscience research, until the latter part of the twentieth century, most clinical neuromodulation efforts involved directly applying electrical current with electrodes, as in ECT.

In 1980, P.A. Merton and H.B. Morton at Queen's Square Hospital in London built a high-voltage electrical stimulator capable of activating muscle directly. This device also stimulated the motor area of the human brain through transcranial electrical stimulation. A brief, high-voltage electric shock over the primary motor cortex produced a brief, mostly synchronous muscle response—the motor-evoked potential (MEP)—and it was immediately apparent that it could be applied for several different purposes (Merton and Morton 1980). However, the use of transcranial electrical stimulation is ultimately limited because it is too painful.

One limitation of electrical stimulation of peripheral nerves is that major nerve trunks contain thousands of fibers with different conduction velocities. Larger-diameter fibers conduct action potentials faster and have lower electrical stimulation thresholds. The decreased current strength with depth below the surface electrodes makes it challenging to stimulate specific fibers selectively. This challenge illustrates an essential difference between electrical and magnetic stimulation. Although electrical current encounters impedance in biological tissue, a magnetic field penetrates various tissues without such resistance.

Recognizing that a pulsed magnetic field does not vary with depth (other than the normal falloff with distance from the coil) and that the induced electrical field remains constant, Anthony Barker and colleagues at the University of Sheffield developed a magnetic peripheral nerve stimulator to address this limitation (Polson et al. 1982). After solving several technical problems, they also showed that it was possible to magnetically stimulate the brain with very little or no pain (Barker et al. 1985).

The discovery by Barker and colleagues generated immediate and widespread interest. Protocols were quickly developed to assess the physiology of the human motor system, including cortical excitability, inhibitory and excitatory mechanisms, conduction time, connectivity, and plasticity. These early experiments found that magnetic stimulation could produce changes in cortical excitability lasting a few seconds or several minutes (Valero-Cabré et al. 2017). Advances in electronics soon allowed for the development of repetitive TMS (rTMS), in which multiple volleys or trains of pulses at frequencies between 1 and 50 Hz can be administered in rapid succession (in this book, *TMS* and *rTMS* are used interchangeably). This technical development allowed magnetic stimulation to induce changes in cortical excitability lasting a few minutes or up to several hours (Camprodon and Pascual-Leone 2016).

Such research yielded important insights, occurring when functional brain imaging studies began to shed light on the pathophysiology of psychiatric disorders. One of the most important findings from this research was *decreased left prefrontal activity in major depression*. Thus, PET and SPECT studies showed a correlation between the depressed state and reduced regional cerebral blood flow and glucose uptake in the left dorsolateral prefrontal cortex (DLPFC) (Mayberg 2003).

In 1995, Mark George and colleagues reported the first clinical application of TMS in treating depression. This open-label study showed that daily stimulation over the left DLPFC significantly improved mood in depressed individuals (George et al. 1995). Similar findings were published a year later (Pascual-Leone et al. 1996) and were soon replicated in a double-blind study (George et al. 1997). These reports sparked years of clinical research, ultimately leading to FDA clearance of the first TMS device to treat depression in 2008.

Basic Principles and Technology of TMS

Principles of Magnetic Stimulation

All TMS devices share the same basic elements (Figure 1–2). A *capacitor* is used to store electricity. A *thyristor switch* is used to precisely control the flow of current. Rapidly turning the current on and off produces a time-varying or moving magnetic field as the current flows through the coil (Davey and Epstein 2000). Peak voltages are typically on the order of 2,000 V, and currents are around 10,000 A. The magnetic field is produced with lines of flux passing perpendicular to the plane of the coil, which is ordinarily placed tangential to the scalp. The magnetic field is as high as 3 teslas and typically lasts about 100 milliseconds. The induced electrical field is orthogonal to the magnetic field and flows in the opposite direction of current flowing in the coil (Hallett 2007).

The size and shape of the TMS *coil* determine the size and shape of the induced electrical field. TMS coils come in many shapes (Figure 1–3). The simplest, and historically the first used for TMS, is a *circular coil* measuring about 8–15 cm in diameter. Such round coils stimulate a large area of the brain but cannot be focused. Two round coils placed side by side form what is known as a *figure-eight* or *butterfly coil*. This design allows stimulation at a more limited and clearly defined location. For this reason, figure-eight coils are widely used for research and therapeutic purposes. Depth of penetration is limited by the laws of physics because magnetic field strength decreases exponentially as a function of distance. The magnetic field strength of TMS is typically 1.5–2.5 teslas at the coil's surface. Although this is about the same strength as a first-generation MRI device and more than 30,000 times stronger than Earth's magnetic field, it is barely detectable only a few centimeters away. Most figure-eight coils activate a cortical area approximately 2–3 cm in diameter and approximately 2–3 cm in depth (Deng et al. 2013). The double-cone coil has deeper penetration but less focus than the figure-eight coil. A newer type

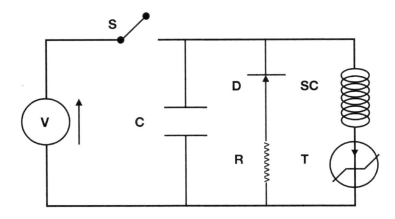

Figure 1–2. Schematic illustration of basic transcranial magnetic stimulation circuit design: capacitor (C), thyristor (T) switch, and stimulating coil (SC).

Ancillary circuits include those for temperature monitoring and for setting the frequency and intensity of pulses. D=diode; R=resistance; S=switch; V=charging circuit.

of coil, the *Hesed* or *H coil*, uses multiple coil windings to achieve even greater penetration depth than the double-cone coil but has even less precise focus as a result. The deeper the penetration is, the more diffuse the electrical field is (see Chapter 9, "Current FDA-Cleared Transcranial Magnetic Stimulation Systems").

Basic Forms of TMS

The three main forms of TMS are single-pulse, paired-pulse, and repetitive TMS, and each produces distinct neurophysiological effects. Typical clinical use of TMS involves repetitive stimulation over some time, but the technology required to do this was not available initially. Thus, early TMS devices delivered only single or paired TMS pulses. Because the motor cortex is so easy to stimulate, most early TMS studies focused primarily on it. These studies provided important insights about the basic physiological effects of TMS and laid the groundwork for later multimodal studies extending TMS investigation beyond the motor cortex.

Note that all TMS is excitatory. Although a given TMS pulse may or may not be strong enough to generate an action potential, all TMS pulses are stimulatory. The terms *excitatory TMS* and *inhibitory TMS*, used in this book and elsewhere, refer to the net modulatory effects on the activity of specific brain regions comprising many neurons. However, all TMS is excitatory at the level of the individual neuron.

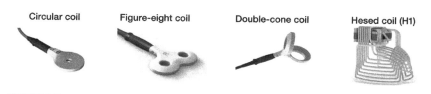

Circular coil   Figure-eight coil   Double-cone coil   Hesed coil (H1)

Figure 1–3. Shapes of transcranial magnetic stimulation coils.

Single-Pulse TMS

Single-pulse TMS is used in motor conduction studies to assess the integrity of the corticospinal tract. A single pulse is applied over the motor cortex, and the MEP of the corresponding contralateral muscle is measured by electromyography. Pathological changes in neurons and synapses are identified by measuring the time between the TMS pulse and the beginning of the MEP.

Single pulses can also determine the motor threshold (MT), which indirectly measures cortical excitability, reflecting the state of neuronal membranes, synapses, and glutamate receptors. The MT is defined as the minimum stimulus intensity needed to induce a muscle contraction in at least 50% of attempts and is expressed as a percentage of the maximum output of the specific TMS device. The MT measured with the muscle at rest, the resting MT, is typically higher than the MT measured with isometric contraction, the active MT. Although typically stable, MT can change with factors that alter cortical excitability (e.g., certain psychotropic medications).

Paired-Pulse TMS

Paired-pulse TMS protocols involve the application of two TMS pulses at different intensities (typically 80% and 120% of the MT) over various time intervals (typically a few milliseconds) to study intracortical inhibition and facilitation. Short-interval cortical inhibition and intracortical facilitation are two widely used protocols. Studies combining these paired-pulse TMS protocols with pharmacology can identify the neurotransmitters involved in these processes.

Short-interval cortical inhibition. Short-interval cortical inhibition involves the application of an initial (conditioning) subthreshold stimulus (unable to elicit an MEP) followed by a second (test) suprathreshold stimulus after a short interval of 1–5 milliseconds. This produces an inhibitory response characterized by reduced MEP amplitude, possibly mediated by $GABA_A$ receptors on cortical interneurons (Camprodon and Pascual-Leone 2016).

Intracortical facilitation. Intracortical facilitation uses the same paired-pulse configuration (a subthreshold conditioning pulse followed by a suprathreshold test pulse) with a longer interstimulus interval of 6–20 milliseconds. This produces an excitatory response characterized by increased MEP amplitude, possibly mediated by glutamate receptors (Camprodon and Pascual-Leone 2016).

In addition to elucidating basic aspects of cortical physiology, similar single- and paired-pulse paradigms, as well as TMS, are used for a variety of clinical applications and research investigations. For example, TMS provides detailed cortical maps to assist with specific neurosurgical procedures. When delivered appropriately in time and space, TMS transiently blocks the function of neuronal networks, creating a time-dependent *virtual lesion* in an otherwise healthy brain.

Although TMS-MEP protocols are extremely helpful in characterizing the neurophysiological properties of the motor cortex, they do not provide direct information about other cortical areas. Combining TMS with a simultaneous electroencephalogram (EEG), however, allows the investigation of excitation, inhibition, and other properties of nonmotor cortical areas with TMS-evoked EEG potentials, as opposed to MEPs.

A complete discussion of this technique is beyond the scope of this book; however, the same modulations of excitability and inhibition induced by TMS stimulation of the motor cortex are observed in other areas of the cortex (Ferrarelli and Phillips 2021). Combined with neuroimaging and pharmacological therapies, TMS of brain regions well beyond the motor cortex indicates that it is a unique and versatile tool for studying the causal relationships between brain activity and behavior (Pascual-Leone 1999).

Repetitive TMS

In contrast to single- and paired-pulse TMS, during which changes in cortical excitability last for only seconds to minutes, rTMS modulates cortical excitability and connectivity by inducing long-term depression–like and long-term potentiation–like changes that outlast the period of stimulation. These effects are parameter dependent. Thus, low-frequency TMS (LF TMS), typically 1 Hz, suppresses activity in the targeted brain region; high-frequency TMS (HF TMS), usually 10–20 Hz, produces excitatory effects.

LF TMS is administered in a continuous train of pulses, whereas HF TMS is administered in trains of specified length separated by specific time intervals (see Figure 1–4). Guidelines regarding the safety of different pulse frequencies and intertrain intervals at varying intensities are designed to limit spreading excitation and decrease the likelihood of seizures

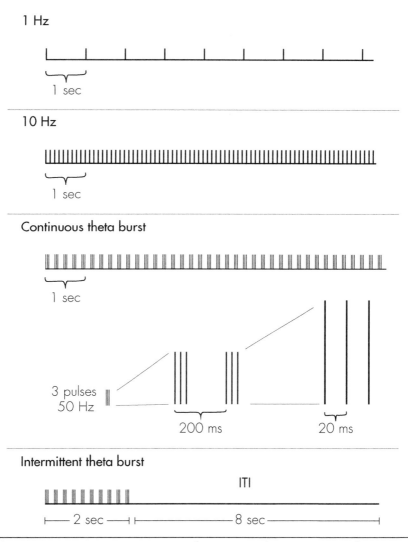

Figure 1–4. Common patterns of transcranial magnetic stimulation (TMS) in clinical settings.

Repetitive TMS (rTMS) involves the application of regularly repeated magnetic pulses; a stimulation rate ≤1 Hz (1 pulse/second) is referred to as low-frequency rTMS, whereas stimulation rates such as 10 Hz (10 pulses/second) are considered high-frequency. Theta burst stimulation (TBS) is a patterned form of TMS in which a three-pulse 50-Hz burst is applied every 200 milliseconds, representing the theta rhythm (5 Hz). Continuous TBS involves an uninterrupted 40-second train for 600 pulses. In intermittent TBS, a 2-second train is delivered every 10 seconds for 600 pulses. ITI=intertrain interval.

Source.   Design and illustration by Cassie Dewey/CDewey Design for Richard A. Bermudes, M.D., August 2024.

(Chen et al. 1997). The original guidelines published in 1998 have been revised twice (Rossi et al. 2009, 2021; Wassermann 1998).

Theta Burst Stimulation

Theta burst stimulation (TBS), a modified TMS protocol, induces differential effects on cortical excitability with greater efficiency (Camprodon and Pascual-Leone 2016). TBS is a patterned form of TMS in which a three-pulse 50-Hz burst is applied every 200 milliseconds, representing the theta rhythm (5 Hz). In intermittent TBS (iTBS), a 2-second train is delivered every 10 seconds for 600 pulses. Continuous TBS (cTBS) involves an uninterrupted 40-second train for 600 pulses (Daskalakis 2014).

iTBS is thought to increase the postsynaptic concentration of calcium ions, an important factor in enhancing synaptic plasticity, and cTBS is believed to decrease this concentration (Huang et al. 2011). Therefore, iTBS produces long-term potentiation–like (excitatory) effects, whereas cTBS produces long-term depression–like (inhibitory) effects on cortical excitability. These neuroplastic changes may occur within seconds (Huang et al. 2005).

TMS Mechanisms of Action

Feelings are mental experiences of body states (Damasio 1999). They may signify physiological needs (e.g., hunger or thirst), tissue responses (e.g., pain or pleasure), threats (e.g., fear or anger), overall function (e.g., malaise or well-being), or social interactions (e.g., obeisance or aggression). In vertebrates, the neural substrates of feelings are found at all levels of the nervous system, from individual neurons to subcortical nuclei and cortical regions. The sophisticated capabilities of the human cerebral cortex, such as memory, language, reasoning, and imagination, allow for more enriched and refined feeling states (emotions) associated with much more complex cognitive and behavioral phenomena. Nevertheless, the underlying physiological substrate is clear. For example, receiving bad news leads to increased blood pressure, irregular heart rhythm, lacrimal secretion (crying), and automatic (unconscious) facial muscle contractions associated with feelings of sadness. Feeling states are inherently subjective and accessible only to those who experience them (Damasio and Carvalho 2013).

The complex and unpleasant human feeling/emotional state known as major depressive disorder is not a unitary disease, but a complex, heterogeneous syndrome that encompasses various symptoms and divergent responses to treatment. Depression may, in fact, consist of multiple syndromes with similar manifestations or phenotypes arising from dysfunction at different levels of biological complexity. From genome to connectome, these levels represent a continuum of increasingly elaborate structures and processes that are grouped into three general categories: those involving a single cell, those involving cell-to-cell communication, and those involving multicellular ensembles that form circuits and networks (Leuchter et al. 2015).

Although distinct physiological functions characterize these categories and levels of organization, they do not operate separately or autonomously. The effects of genetic and molecular factors are translated from the bottom up and influence the clinical phenotype, whereas the influence of anatomical and functional networks is translated from the top down and affects cellular communication and intracellular processes.

In a similar manner, treatments for depression exert a range of effects at multiple levels. Thus, understanding the mechanism of action of TMS is approached from both top-down and bottom-up perspectives, including the molecular level (e.g., genes and neurotransmitters); the synaptic level (e.g., neuroplastic changes); higher-level cortical function (e.g., metabolism and electrophysiology); and the brain-body interaction as a whole (e.g., autonomic nervous system). Through multiple methods of investigation, much is now known. In this section, we highlight key findings from these diverse approaches, specifically focusing on understanding TMS as a potential treatment approach.

Gene Effects

TMS affects the expression of specific stress response genes and genetic polymorphisms, which may dictate TMS response. *C-FOS* is an immediate early response gene used as a marker of neuronal activity. It is associated with several neural and behavioral events, including the acute stress response (Velazquez et al. 2015). LF TMS reduces *C-FOS* expression (Teyssier et al. 2013). The brain-derived neurotrophic factor gene *BDNF* is one of many thought to influence synaptic plasticity. The Val/Val genotype is associated with greater susceptibility to TMS-induced plasticity than the Val/Met genotype (Cheeran et al. 2008). Results from TMS studies examining polymorphisms in the genes that code for the serotonin transporter promoter region (SERTPR), the serotonin type 1A (5-HT$_{1A}$) receptor promoter region (−1019C/G) (Zanardi et al. 2007), and catechol O-methyltransferase (COMT) (Malaguti et al. 2011) are inconsistent. Thus, to date, no genotype predictors of TMS response have been clearly identified.

Neurotransmitter Effects

TMS affects neurotransmitter activity in multiple brain regions. HF TMS increases glutamate in the stimulated region. Magnetic resonance spectroscopy demonstrates a sustained increase in prefrontal glutamate levels correlated with antidepressant response (Luborzewski et al. 2007). A SPECT study found increased bilateral DLPFC 5-HT$_{2A}$ binding and decreased right hippocampus 5-HT$_{2A}$ binding in HF TMS responders (Baeken et al. 2011). Other imaging studies reported increased dopamine binding in the ipsilateral caudate nucleus (Strafella et al. 2001) and decreased binding in the striatum (Pogarell et al. 2006); increased norepinephrine in the locus coeruleus (Yukimasa et al. 2006); increased acetylcholine in the basal forebrain and striatum (Luborzewski et al. 2007); and increased GABA in the medial PFC, hippocampus, and striatum (Bajbouj et al. 2005; Dubin et al. 2016). Although TMS alters neurotransmitter levels and turnover in widely distributed brain regions, the precise clinical significance of these changes remains uncertain.

Metabolic Effects

TMS affects metabolism in a wide range of cortical and subcortical regions. Various methods have been used to investigate the effects of TMS on brain metabolism, including SPECT, PET, functional MRI, and functional near-infrared spectroscopy. These studies documented that TMS produces widespread changes in brain metabolism with important lateralized and frequency-dependent variables (Catafau et al. 2001). Thus, left prefrontal TMS produces a different pattern of changes from right prefrontal TMS (laterality effect), and HF TMS produces a different pattern of changes from LF TMS (frequency effect).

HF TMS applied to either hemisphere increases regional cerebral blood flow in the stimulated region (Knoch et al. 2006) and in other trans-synaptically linked areas, including the ipsilateral cingulate cortex, amygdala, bilateral hippocampus, thalamus, and cerebellum. However, the specific linked areas differ from left to right (Speer et al. 2000). LF TMS applied to either hemisphere decreases activity at the stimulation site and in the mirror contralateral cortical region (Kozel et al. 2009). LF TMS over the left DLPFC affects the same areas as HF TMS over the right DLPFC, suggesting a laterality-frequency interaction. In general, HF TMS increases left DLPFC activity, and LF TMS decreases right DLPFC activity. It also may be said that all TMS is bilateral TMS because unilateral TMS can have transhemispheric effects, modulating the activity and connectivity of regions in both the simulated hemisphere and the contralateral (nonstimulated) hemisphere.

Electrophysiological Effects

TMS affects EEG power (i.e., the strength and intensity of the brain's oscillatory patterns within specific frequency bands) across multiple frequencies. EEG studies of depression often focus on alpha activity in the PFC, which is negatively correlated with metabolic activity (Cook et al. 1998). Studies consistently show increased alpha power on the left, indicating hypoactivity, whereas the right PFC demonstrates decreased alpha power, indicating hyperactivity (Henriques and Davidson 1991). This frontal alpha asymmetry is well established. Asymmetrical slow delta wave activity is seen in the frontotemporal area along with decreased interhemispheric coherence in delta and theta bands (Lieber 1988), as well as increased right-sided delta and theta activity (Kwon et al. 1996).

HF TMS produces more significant and more widespread electrophysiological changes compared with low-frequency stimulation. HF TMS increases alpha, theta, and delta power in central and parietal areas. LF TMS produces similar effects on alpha and theta power but diminishes delta power in the left frontal and temporal regions (Valiulis et al. 2012). Although left-sided HF TMS and right-sided LF TMS were equally effective in large population studies (Chen et al. 2013), these findings suggest that alpha asymmetry and delta power differences between the hemispheres serve as markers in choosing the most effective TMS protocol for a given patient.

Neuroendocrine Effects

TMS may normalize activity of the hypothalamic-pituitary-adrenal (HPA) axis. Hyperactivity of this axis is seen in many patients with depression, along with a positive correlation between symptom severity and increased cortisol release (Pariante and Miller 2001). The HPA axis involves a complex set of direct interactions and reciprocal loops of negative feedback between the frontal cortex, including the DLPFC, and the subgenual anterior cingulate cortex (sgACC), hypothalamus, pituitary gland, and adrenal gland. TMS over the left DLPFC decreases cortisol levels (Baeken et al. 2009) and can normalize cortisol release induced by the dexamethasone suppression test (Reid and Pridmore 1999). Glucocorticoid receptors in the sgACC play a crucial role in the negative feedback loop of cortisol secretion during stress. Increased sgACC activity may contribute to excess cortisol secretion in depression (Diorio et al. 1993). TMS modulates activity in interconnected brain regions with high-density glucocorticoid receptors, including the sgACC and the DLPFC. The suppression of depressive symptoms is greater when targeting the area in the left DLPFC with the most anticorrelated connectivity in the sgACC (Fox et al. 2012).

However, HPA axis abnormalities do not occur in all patients with depression (Schutter and van Honk 2010). In terms of other possible endocrine effects, applying TMS did not affect levels of thyroid-stimulating hormone, thyroxine, prolactin, estrogen, or testosterone (Meille et al. 2017).

Autonomic Nervous System Effects

TMS may increase the activity of the parasympathetic nervous system. There are case reports of TMS-induced vasovagal syncope (e.g., Kesar et al. 2016). This rare, but benign, adverse effect may be accompanied by myoclonic jerks, causing it to be confused with a seizure at times. The mechanism underlying these events is uncertain, but the fact that they occur indicates that TMS affects vagal tone. Autonomic regulation of the cardiovascular system involves several regions in the so-called central autonomic network, including the PFC, sgACC, and amygdala (Benarroch 1993). Through vagal (i.e., parasympathetic) activation, the PFC may produce a parasympathetic inhibitory influence on subcortical nodes in this network (Thayer and Lane 2009). Depression is associated with reduced prefrontal parasympathetic inhibition (Kidwell and Ellenbroek 2018). Prefrontal TMS reduces heart rate, suggesting efferent stimulation of the frontal vagal network involved in cardiovascular control (Makovac et al. 2017). Both implantable and transcutaneous auricular vagus nerve stimulation may treat depression, possibly through afferent stimulation of the solitary nucleus of the medulla, median dorsal raphe nucleus, and locus coeruleus through serotonergic and noradrenergic mechanisms (e.g., Austelle et al. 2022). TMS may produce similar effects through this mechanism of action, but the significance of its modulation of vagus nerve activity in treating depression remains uncertain.

Immune System Effects

TMS may directly or indirectly influence immune function and inflammation. Animal studies found that TMS reduces glial activation, decreases apoptosis, and improves functional recovery after focal brain injury (Sasso et al. 2016). These studies also suggested that TMS reduces levels of several markers of inflammation and may influence the gut microbiome in a top-down manner, possibly by stimulating descending pathways (Seewoo et al. 2022). Human studies also reported that TMS modulates gut microbiome composition, perhaps through norepinephrine mechanisms, reducing obesity-associated microbiome variations and promoting bacterial species with anti-inflammatory properties.

The inflammatory reflex is a vagus nerve–based neural circuit in which afferent nerve signaling activated by inflammatory mediators, such as cytokines and pathogen-derived molecular signals, leads to efferent vagal activity that dampens pro-inflammatory cytokine production (Tynan et al. 2022). In patients with poststroke depression, TMS significantly reduced levels of several serum inflammatory factors, including interleukin 1β and tumor necrosis factor α, possibly through vagal pathways (Liu et al. 2022). Investigation into the use of TMS and other forms of noninvasive brain stimulation to modulate the immune reflex is still in its infancy, and the clinical significance of these early findings is uncertain (Perrin and Pariante 2020).

Neuroplastic Effects

TMS alters synaptic plasticity and promotes neurogenesis. Cellular models of learning and memory involve multiple mechanisms, including the remodeling of synaptic spines (Holtmaat and Svoboda 2009), upregulation of transcription factors (Alberini 2009), adult neurogenesis (Aimone et al. 2014), epigenetic remodeling through DNA methylation (Jiang et al. 2008), and the effects of neurotrophic factors (Chen et al. 2010). Similar mechanisms leading to enhanced synaptic plasticity may be part of the shared mechanism of action of all effective antidepressant treatments (Racagni and Popoli 2008).

TMS increases the expression and signaling of *BDNF*, which mediates neuroplasticity in the hippocampus and cortex (Dall'Agnol et al. 2014). In this context, TMS enhances neuroplasticity in cortical and corticospinal systems, possibly through changes in *BDNF* release and expression (Esslinger et al. 2014). Downstream effects of *BDNF* on synaptic neuroplasticity and neurogenesis, particularly in the hippocampus, are thought to play an essential role in TMS treatment of depression (Duman and Aghajanian 2012). The clinical impact of TMS effects on neuroplasticity remains under investigation.

Neural Network Effects

The human brain consists of multiple distinct and interacting networks. Investigating these networks provides a systematic framework for understanding the brain's organization and function in healthy and diseased states (Bressler and Menon 2010). Research using advanced neuroimaging methods, such as PET and functional MRI, has identified networks underlying processes such as self-reflection, perception, and attention. These include the central executive network (CEN), default mode network (DMN), and salience network (SN) (Figure 1–5; Williams 2016).

Neuropsychiatric disorders are increasingly conceptualized as *network disorders* characterized by altered activity within and between distinct functional networks. Thus, brain network interrelationships with each other and their component neurocircuits are not static and can change as a function of internal and external demands (Cocchi et al. 2018). These ongoing dynamic activity patterns can rearrange connectivity between various circuits within and across networks, altering their interactions. Of note, this changeability may also help to explain some of the response variability in previous clinical studies of TMS for psychiatric disorders (e.g., major depressive disorder, OCD).

Attention has focused on the DMN, SN, and CEN (e.g., Liston et al. 2014). For example, in major depression, connectivity abnormalities between the sgACC (an essential node of the DMN) and the DLPFC (part of the SN and CEN) have been identified (Pizzagalli 2011) (see Chapter 2, "Transcranial Magnetic Stimulation Therapy for Major Depression"). Similarly, most TMS trials in OCD have targeted frontal and prefrontal brain regions encompassing frontostriatal networks (Cocchi et al. 2018) (see Chapter 6, "Transcranial Magnetic Stimulation for OCD"). For TMS to modulate a network implicated in a neuropsychiatric condition, a cortical or subcortical target must not be too distal from the scalp's surface so that it is within the magnetic field.

One particular set of cortical and subcortical structures, which includes the DLPFC, medial PFC, orbitofrontal cortex, sgACC, insula, thalamus, hypothalamus, and hippocampus, constitutes a discrete *cortico-striatal-thalamic-cortical (CSTC) loop*. The dorsal ACC and the anterior insula constitute the core of the SN and are a critical hub within the brain's functional architecture at the intersection of cognitive, affective, and somatosensory processing (Downar et al. 2016). Thus, this CSTC loop is particularly relevant to understanding the pathophysiology of several neuropsychiatric conditions and TMS treatment response.

Specific brain oscillatory patterns within the CSTC loop characterize awake resting state (e.g., eyes-closed alpha and eyes-open beta activity); sleep stages (e.g., K-complexes and sleep spindles); and perceptual, motor, and cognitive states. Changes in these oscillatory patterns may represent a common mechanism in various neuropsychiatric disorders, including depression (Llinás et al. 1999). In this model of thalamocortical dysrhyth-

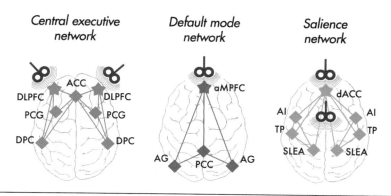

Figure 1–5. Brain distinct and interacting networks underlying processes such as self-reflection, perception, and attention: central executive network, default mode network, and salience network.

The default mode network encompasses the anterior medial prefrontal cortex (aMPFC), posterior cingulate cortex (PCC), and angular gyrus (AG). This network comes into play when the brain is at rest or when individuals are prompted to contemplate their self-generated thoughts in task-free circumstances.

The salience network, identified by key nodes in the dorsal anterior cingulate cortex (dACC), anterior insula (AI), and sublenticular extended amygdala (SLEA), is crucial for detecting significant environmental changes. These changes can be both internal and external, signaling the necessity for cognitive control.

The central executive network, comprising the dorsolateral PFC (DLPFC; includes the anterior PFC and inferior frontal cortex), ACC, dorsal parietal cortex (DPC), and precentral gyrus (PCG), and their interconnectivity, supports higher cognitive functions such as working memory, cognitive flexibility, and selective attention.

TP=temporal pole.

Source. Design and illustration by Cassie Dewey/CDewey Design for Richard A. Bermudes, M.D., August 2024.

mia, resting-state alpha activity (8–12 Hz) slows down to theta frequencies (4–8 Hz) and is associated with an increase in surrounding beta and gamma (25–50 Hz) activity (Vanneste et al. 2018).

One immediate effect of HF TMS is the synchronization or entrainment of oscillations in the targeted area to the frequency of the stimulating magnet (Fuggetta et al. 2008). This oscillatory entrainment to the stimulation frequency is not sustained. However, once stimulation has ceased, TMS enhances the emergence of the natural, intrinsic rhythms of the stimulated area (Rosanova et al. 2009). These oscillatory changes may contribute to enhanced plasticity in the stimulated area and the rapid spread of the reemerging natural rhythms to multiple interconnected limbic structures. Evidence, therefore, suggests that TMS may act in a top-down manner by reducing abnormal low-frequency resonance in thalamo-cortical loops, thereby facilitating the reemergence of normal endogenous rhythms to *reset* oscillatory circuits, normal brain network function, and the processes that regulate normal mood (Leuchter et al. 2015).

Thalamocortical dysrhythmia is implicated in other neuropsychiatric disorders, including OCD, Parkinson's disease, tinnitus, and central pain syndromes, all of which show some evidence of response to TMS. Because a variety of neurochemical and ionic mechanisms govern both the firing pattern of individual neurons and the resonant oscillatory frequency of neuronal circuits, antidepressant medication can act in a bottom-up man-ner to resolve thalamocortical dysrhythmia at the cellular level through effects on voltage-gated ion channels (Rammes and Rupprecht 2007). In addition to TMS, other antidepressant treatments (e.g., psychotherapy, ECT, vagus nerve stimulation, and ketamine) have been reported to nor-malize DLPFC and sgACC activity (Gyurak et al. 2016), perhaps through mechanisms that also restore normal CSTC rhythms.

Conclusion

TMS is a noninvasive technique for stimulating the human brain using a high-strength pulsed magnetic field, which reliably induces electrical fields in circumscribed cortical regions in accordance with Faraday's law of induction. TMS constitutes a significant advance in the noninvasive study of human brain function and is used as a probe to delineate and study both normal and dysfunctional neural networks.

TMS is best conceptualized as a *circuit and network modulator* with clinical effects depending on how the stimulation is applied and propa-gated through the particular brain circuit or network. TMS pulses are administered in different ways to produce temporary and long-lasting neuroplastic changes in brain function. Effective clinical application of TMS requires the identification of a relevant and accessible cortical target and use of the requisite pulse parameters to induce the intended neuro-plastic changes and associated clinical benefits.

Improvements in TMS technology, such as the development of new stimulation coils, and modifications in TMS technique, including the use of different pulse parameters such as TBS, will enhance TMS's efficiency and clinical efficacy. In addition, several cortical sites other than the DLPFC are potential therapeutic targets.

Although the mechanisms of action of TMS are not fully understood, evidence suggests that its therapeutic effects are the result of neuroplastic changes in specific brain networks and corticolimbic circuits involved in the phenotypic expression of core symptoms of major depression and other psychiatric disorders. These findings, together with those derived from different lines of research (e.g., neuroimaging), shed light on the pathophysiology and circuit and/or network dysfunction associated with other neuropsychiatric disorders (e.g., OCD, schizophrenia, and PTSD), leading to clinical applications beyond major depression and other major mood syndromes.

KEY POINTS

- Transcranial magnetic stimulation (TMS) is a noninvasive neuro-modulation method with a growing range of diagnostic and therapeutic applications.

- TMS targets specific areas of the cerebral cortex but produces measurable changes in distal cortical and subcortical areas, translating to changes in dysfunctional brain networks implicated in neuropsychiatric conditions.

- TMS produces physiological changes at multiple levels of the nervous system and in other organ systems.

- Clinical effects of TMS depend on multiple parameters, such as stimulus target, frequency, and intensity.

References

Aimone JB, Li Y, Lee SW, et al: Regulation and function of adult neurogenesis: from genes to cognition. Physiol Rev 94(4):991–1026, 2014 25287858

Alberini CM: Transcription factors in long-term memory and synaptic plasticity. Physiol Rev 89(1):121–145, 2009 19126756

Austelle CW, O'Leary GH, Thompson S, et al: A comprehensive review of vagus nerve stimulation for depression. Neuromodulation 25(3):309–315, 2022 35396067

Baeken C, De Raedt R, Leyman L, et al: The impact of one HF-rTMS session on mood and salivary cortisol in treatment resistant unipolar melancholic depressed patients. J Affect Disord 113(1–2):100–108, 2009 18571733

Baeken C, De Raedt R, Bossuyt A, et al: The impact of HF-rTMS treatment on serotonin(2A) receptors in unipolar melancholic depression. Brain Stimul 4(2):104–111, 2011 21511211

Bajbouj M, Brakemeier EL, Schubert F, et al: Repetitive transcranial magnetic stimulation of the dorsolateral prefrontal cortex and cortical excitability in patients with major depressive disorder. Exp Neurol 196(2):332–338, 2005 16194530

Barker AT, Jalinous R, Freeston IL: Non-invasive magnetic stimulation of human motor cortex. Lancet 1(8437):1106–1107, 1985 2860322

Benarroch EE: The central autonomic network: functional organization, dysfunction, and perspective. Mayo Clin Proc 68(10):988–1001, 1993

Bressler SL, Menon V: Large-scale brain networks in cognition: emerging methods and principles. Trends Cogn Sci 14(6):277–290, 2010 20493761

Camprodon JA, Pascual-Leone A: Multimodal applications of transcranial magnetic stimulation for circuit-based psychiatry. JAMA Psychiatry 73(4):407–408, 2016 26981644

Catafau AM, Perez V, Gironell A, et al: SPECT mapping of cerebral activity changes induced by repetitive transcranial magnetic stimulation in depressed patients: a pilot study. Psychiatry Res 106(3):151–160, 2001 11382537

Cheeran B, Talelli P, Mori F, et al: A common polymorphism in the brain-derived neurotrophic factor gene (BDNF) modulates human cortical plasticity and the response to rTMS. J Physiol 586(23):5717–5725, 2008 18845611

Chen J, Zhou C, Wu B, et al: Left versus right repetitive transcranial magnetic stimulation in treating major depression: a meta-analysis of randomised controlled trials. Psychiatry Res 210:1260–1264, 2013

Chen LY, Rex CS, Sanaiha Y, et al: Learning induces neurotrophin signaling at hippocampal synapses. Proc Natl Acad Sci U S A 107(15):7030–7035, 2010 20356829

Chen R, Gerloff C, Classen J, et al: Safety of different inter-train intervals for repetitive transcranial magnetic stimulation and recommendations for safe ranges of stimulation parameters. Electroencephalogr Clin Neurophysiol 105(6):415–421, 1997 9448642

Cocchi L, Zalesky A, Nott Z et al: Transcranial magnetic stimulation in obsessive-compulsive disorder: a focus on network mechanisms and state dependence. Neuroimage Clin 19:661–674, 2018 30023172

Cook IA, O'Hara R, Uijtdehaage SH, et al: Assessing the accuracy of topographic EEG mapping for determining local brain function. Electroencephalogr Clin Neurophysiol 107(6):408–414, 1998 9922086

Dall'Agnol L, Medeiros LF, Torres IL, et al: Repetitive transcranial magnetic stimulation increases the corticospinal inhibition and the brain-derived neurotrophic factor in chronic myofascial pain syndrome: an explanatory double-blinded, randomized, sham-controlled trial. J Pain 15(8):845–855, 2014 24865417

Damasio A: The Feeling of What Happens: Body and Emotion in the Making of Consciousness. New York, Harcourt, 1999

Damasio A, Carvalho GB: The nature of feelings: evolutionary and neurobiological origins. Nat Rev Neurosci 14(2):143–152, 2013 23329161

Daskalakis ZJ: Theta-burst transcranial magnetic stimulation in depression: when less may be more. Brain 137(Pt 7):1860–1862, 2014 24833712

Davey K, Epstein CM: Magnetic stimulation coil and circuit design. IEEE Trans Biomed Eng 47(11):1493–1499, 2000 11077743

Deng ZD, Lisanby SH, Peterchev AV: Electric field depth-focality tradeoff in transcranial magnetic stimulation: simulation comparison of 50 coil designs. Brain Stimul 6(1):1–13, 2013 22483681

Diorio D, Viau V, Meaney MJ: The role of the medial prefrontal cortex (cingulate gyrus) in the regulation of hypothalamic-pituitary-adrenal responses to stress. J Neurosci 13(9):3839–3847, 1993 8396170

Downar J, Blumberger DM, Daskalakis ZJ: The neural crossroads of psychiatric illness: an emerging target for brain stimulation. Trends Cogn Sci 20(2):107–120, 2016 26655436

Dubin MJ, Mao X, Banerjee S, et al: Elevated prefrontal cortex GABA in patients with major depressive disorder after TMS treatment measured with proton magnetic resonance spectroscopy. J Psychiatry Neurosci 41(3):E37–E45, 2016 26900793

Duman RS, Aghajanian GK: Synaptic dysfunction in depression: potential therapeutic targets. Science 338(6103):68–72, 2012 23042884

Esslinger C, Schüler N, Sauer C, et al: Induction and quantification of prefrontal cortical network plasticity using 5 Hz rTMS and fMRI. Hum Brain Mapp 35(1):140–151, 2014 22965696

Faraday M: Effects on the production of electricity from magnetism (1831), in Michael Faraday. Edited by Williams LP. New York, Basic Books, 1965, p 531

Ferrarelli F, Phillips ML: Examining and modulating neural circuits in psychiatric disorders with transcranial magnetic stimulation and electroencephalography: present practices and future developments. Am J Psychiatry 178(5):400–413, 2021 33653120

Fox MD, Buckner RL, White MP, et al: Efficacy of transcranial magnetic stimulation targets for depression is related to intrinsic functional connectivity with the subgenual cingulate. Biol Psychiatry 72(7):595–603, 2012 22658708

Fuggetta G, Pavone EF, Fiaschi A, et al: Acute modulation of cortical oscillatory activities during short trains of high-frequency repetitive transcranial magnetic stimulation of the human motor cortex: a combined EEG and TMS study. Hum Brain Mapp 29(1):1–13, 2008 17318833

George MS, Wassermann EM, Williams WA, et al: Daily repetitive transcranial magnetic stimulation (rTMS) improves mood in depression. Neuroreport 6(14):1853–1856, 1995 8547583

George MS, Wassermann EM, Kimbrell TA, et al: Mood improvement following daily left prefrontal repetitive transcranial magnetic stimulation in patients with depression: a placebo-controlled crossover trial. Am J Psychiatry 154(12):1752–1756, 1997 9396958

Gyurak A, Patenaude B, Korgaonkar MS, et al: Frontoparietal activation during response inhibition predicts remission to antidepressants in patients with major depression. Biol Psychiatry 79(4):274–281, 2016 25891220

Hallett M: Transcranial magnetic stimulation: a primer. Neuron 55(2):187–199, 2007 17640522

Henriques JB, Davidson RJ: Left frontal hypoactivation in depression. J Abnorm Psychol 100(4):535–545, 1991 1757667

Holtmaat A, Svoboda K: Experience-dependent structural synaptic plasticity in the mammalian brain. Nat Rev Neurosci 10(9):647–658, 2009 19693029

Huang YZ, Edwards MJ, Rounis E, et al: Theta burst stimulation of the human motor cortex. Neuron 45(2):201–206, 2005 15664172

Huang YZ, Rothwell JC, Chen RS, et al: The theoretical model of theta burst form of repetitive transcranial magnetic stimulation. Clin Neurophysiol 122(5):1011–1018, 2011 20869307

Jiang Y, Langley B, Lubin FD, et al: Epigenetics in the nervous system. J Neurosci 28(46):11753–11759, 2008 19005036

Kesar TM, McDonald HS, Eicholtz SP, et al: Case report of syncope during a single pulse transcranial magnetic stimulation experiment in a healthy adult participant. Brain Stimul 9(3):471–472, 2016 27050115

Kidwell M, Ellenbroek BA: Heart and soul: heart rate variability and major depression. Behav Pharmacol 29(2 and 3 Spec Issue):152–164, 2018 29543649

Knoch D, Treyer V, Regard M, et al: Lateralized and frequency-dependent effects of prefrontal rTMS on regional cerebral blood flow. Neuroimage 31(2):641–648, 2006 16497518

Kozel FA, Tian F, Dhamne S, et al: Using simultaneous repetitive transcranial magnetic stimulation/functional near infrared spectroscopy (rTMS/fNIRS) to measure brain activation and connectivity. Neuroimage 47(4):1177–1184, 2009 19446635

Kwon JS, Youn T, Jung HY: Right hemisphere abnormalities in major depression: quantitative electroencephalographic findings before and after treatment. J Affect Disord 40(3):169–173, 1996 8897116

Leuchter AF, Hunter AM, Krantz DE, et al: Rhythms and blues: modulation of oscillatory synchrony and the mechanism of action of antidepressant treatments. Ann N Y Acad Sci 1344(1):78–91, 2015 25809789

Lieber AL: Diagnosis and subtyping of depressive disorders by quantitative electroencephalography, II: interhemispheric measures are abnormal in major depressives and frequency analysis may discriminate certain subtypes. Hillside J Clin Psychiatry 10(1):84–97, 1988 3410406

Liston C, Chen AC, Zebley BD, et al: Default mode network mechanisms of transcranial magnetic stimulation in depression. Biol Psychiatry 76(7):517–526, 2014 24629537

Liu S, Wang X, Yu R, et al: Effect of transcranial magnetic stimulation on treatment effect and immune function. Saudi J Biol Sci 29(1):379–384, 2022 35002433

Llinás RR, Ribary U, Jeanmonod D, et al: Thalamocortical dysrhythmia: a neurological and neuropsychiatric syndrome characterized by magnetoencephalography. Proc Natl Acad Sci U S A 96(26):15222–15227, 1999 10611366

Luborzewski A, Schubert F, Seifert F, et al: Metabolic alterations in the dorsolateral prefrontal cortex after treatment with high-frequency repetitive transcranial magnetic stimulation in patients with unipolar major depression. J Psychiatr Res 41(7):606–615, 2007 16600298

Makovac E, Thayer JF, Ottaviani C: A meta-analysis of non-invasive brain stimulation and autonomic functioning: implications for brain-heart pathways to cardiovascular disease. Neurosci Biobehav Rev 74(Pt B):330–341, 2017 27185286

Malaguti A, Rossini D, Lucca A, et al: Role of COMT, 5-HT(1A), and SERT genetic polymorphisms on antidepressant response to transcranial magnetic stimulation. Depress Anxiety 28(7):568–573, 2011 21449006

Mayberg HS: Modulating dysfunctional limbic-cortical circuits in depression: towards development of brain-based algorithms for diagnosis and optimised treatment. Br Med Bull 65(1):193–207, 2003 12697626

Meille V, Verges B, Lalanne L, et al: Effects of transcranial magnetic stimulation on the hypothalamic-pituitary axis in depression: results of a pilot study. J Neuropsychiatry Clin Neurosci 29(1):70–73, 2017 27539376

Merton PA, Morton HB: Stimulation of the cerebral cortex in the intact human subject. Nature 285(5762):227, 1980 7374773

Pariante CM, Miller AH: Glucocorticoid receptors in major depression: relevance to pathophysiology and treatment. Biol Psychiatry 49(5):391–404, 2001 11274650

Pascual-Leone A: Transcranial magnetic stimulation: studying the brain-behaviour relationship by induction of "virtual lesions." Philos Trans R Soc Lond B Biol Sci 354(1387):1229–1238, 1999 10466148

Pascual-Leone A, Rubio B, Pallardó F, et al: Rapid-rate transcranial magnetic stimulation of left dorsolateral prefrontal cortex in drug-resistant depression. Lancet 348(9022):233–237, 1996 8684201

Perrin AJ, Pariante CM: Endocrine and immune effects of non-convulsive neuro-stimulation in depression: a systematic review. Brain Behav Immun 87:910–920, 2020 32126288

Pizzagalli DA: Frontocingulate dysfunction in depression: toward biomarkers of treatment response. Neuropsychopharmacology 36(1):183–206, 2011 20861828

Pogarell O, Koch W, Pöpperl G, et al: Striatal dopamine release after prefrontal repetitive transcranial magnetic stimulation in major depression: preliminary results of a dynamic [123I] IBZM SPECT study. J Psychiatr Res 40(4):307–314, 2006 16259998

Polson MJR, Barker AT, Freeston IL: Stimulation of nerve trunks with time-varying magnetic fields. Med Biol Eng Comput 20(2):243–244, 1982 7098583

Racagni G, Popoli M: Cellular and molecular mechanisms in the long-term action of antidepressants. Dialogues Clin Neurosci 10(4):385–400, 2008 19170396

Rammes G, Rupprecht R: Modulation of ligand-gated ion channels by antidepres-sants and antipsychotics. Mol Neurobiol 35(2):160–174, 2007 17917105

Reid PD, Pridmore S: Dexamethasone suppression test reversal in rapid transcra-nial magnetic stimulation-treated depression. Aust N Z J Psychiatry 33(2):274–277, 1999 10336227

Rosanova M, Casali A, Bellina V, et al: Natural frequencies of human corticotha-lamic circuits. J Neurosci 29(24):7679–7685, 2009 19535579

Rossi S, Hallett M, Rossini PM, et al: Safety, ethical considerations, and applica-tion guidelines for the use of transcranial magnetic stimulation in clinical practice and research. Clin Neurophysiol 120(12):2008–2039, 2009 19833552

Rossi S, Antal A, Bestmann S, et al: Safety and recommendations for TMS use in healthy subjects and patient populations, with updates on training, ethical and regulatory issues: expert guidelines. Clin Neurophysiol 132(1):269–306, 2021 33243615

Sasso V, Bisicchia E, Latini L, et al: Repetitive transcranial magnetic stimulation reduces remote apoptotic cell death and inflammation after focal brain in-jury. J Neuroinflammation 13(1):150, 2016 27301743

Schutter DJ, van Honk J: An endocrine perspective on the role of steroid hor-mones in the antidepressant treatment efficacy of transcranial magnetic stim-ulation. Psychoneuroendocrinology 35(1):171–178, 2010 19443126

Seewoo BJ, Chua EG, Arena-Foster Y, et al: Changes in the rodent gut micro-biome following chronic restraint stress and low-intensity rTMS. Neurobiol Stress 17:100430, 2022 35146078

Speer AM, Kimbrell TA, Wassermann EM, et al: Opposite effects of high and low frequency rTMS on regional brain activity in depressed patients. Biol Psychiatry 48(12):1133–1141, 2000 11137053

Strafella AP, Paus T, Barrett J, et al: Repetitive transcranial magnetic stimulation of the human prefrontal cortex induces dopamine release in the caudate nucleus. J Neurosci 21(15):RC157, 2001 11459878

Teyssier JR, Trojak B, Chauvet-Gelinier JC, et al: Low frequency transcranial magnetic stimulation downregulates expression of stress genes in blood leucocytes: preliminary evidence. J Psychiatr Res 47(7):935–936, 2013 23548330

Thayer JF, Lane RD: Claude Bernard and the heart-brain connection: further elaboration of a model of neurovisceral integration. Neurosci Biobehav Rev 33(2):81–88, 2009 18771686

Theodore WH: Book review: Handbook of Transcranial Magnetic Stimulation. Edited by A. Pascual-Leone, N.J. Davey, J. Rothwell, E.M. Wasseran, B.K. Puri, Arnold, London, 2001. £110 sterling, ISBN 0340720093. Epilepsy Behav 3(4):404, 2002

Thompson SP: A physiological effect of an alternating magnetic field. Proc R Soc Lond B 82(557):396–398, 1910

Tynan A, Brines M, Chavan SS: Control of inflammation using non-invasive neuromodulation: past, present and promise. Int Immunol 34(2):119–128, 2022 34558623

Valero-Cabré A, Amengual JL, Stengel C, et al: Transcranial magnetic stimulation in basic and clinical neuroscience: a comprehensive review of fundamental principles and novel insights. Neurosci Biobehav Rev 83:381–404, 2017 29032089

Valiulis V, Gerulskis G, Dapšys K, et al: Electrophysiological differences between high and low frequency rTMS protocols in depression treatment. Acta Neurobiol Exp (Wars) 72(3):283–295, 2012 23093015

Vanneste S, Song JJ, De Ridder D: Thalamocortical dysrhythmia detected by machine learning. Nat Commun 9(1):1103, 2018 29549239

Velazquez FN, Caputto BL, Boussin FD: c-Fos importance for brain development. Aging (Albany NY) 7(12):1028–1029, 2015 26684501

Wassermann EM: Risk and safety of repetitive transcranial magnetic stimulation: report and suggested guidelines from the International Workshop on the Safety of Repetitive Transcranial Magnetic Stimulation, June 5–7, 1996. Electroencephalogr Clin Neurophysiol 108(1):1–16, 1998 9474057

Williams LM: Precision psychiatry: a neural circuit taxonomy for depression and anxiety. Lancet Psychiatry 3(5):472–480, 2016 27150382

Yukimasa T, Yoshimura R, Tamagawa A, et al: High-frequency repetitive transcranial magnetic stimulation improves refractory depression by influencing catecholamine and brain-derived neurotrophic factors. Pharmacopsychiatry 39(2):52–59, 2006 16555165

Zanardi R, Magri L, Rossini D, et al: Role of serotonergic gene polymorphisms on response to transcranial magnetic stimulation in depression. Eur Neuropsychopharmacol 17(10):651–657, 2007 17466494

2

Transcranial Magnetic Stimulation Therapy for Major Depression

Karl I. Lanocha, M.D.
Richard A. Bermudes, M.D.
Philip G. Janicak, M.D.

Major depressive disorder (MDD) is one of the most disabling conditions globally. The World Health Organization (2023) estimates that more than 280 million people worldwide have depression. Lifetime prevalence varies by region, ranging from 10% to 20%, depending on population demographics and methodologies (Hasin et al. 2018; Lim et al. 2018). MDD imposes substantial economic burdens, with the financial cost of MDD in the United States reaching $326 billion by 2020, a 38% increase from 2010 levels (Greenberg et al. 2021).

Despite available treatments, 50%–70% of individuals with depression either partially respond or do not respond at all to antidepressants and augmentation agents (Pigott et al. 2023; Rush et al. 2020). Treatment-resistant depression (TRD) (Fava and Davidson 1996) is associated with higher disability, morbidity, and mortality (Greden 2001).

Zhdanava et al. (2021) calculated that the total annual burden of medication-treated MDD in the United States was $92.7 billion, with $43.8 billion (47.2%) attributed to TRD. They found that TRD contributed to 56.6% of the health care burden, 47.7% of the unemployment burden, and 32.2% of the productivity burden of medication-treated MDD.

Suicide remains a major concern among those with MDD, because patients experience a 20-fold increase in suicide risk and a 2-fold increase in all-cause mortality (Nordentoft et al. 2019). The lifetime suicide risk for individuals with depression is estimated to be between 2% and 4% (Nordentoft et al. 2019).

In clinical settings, the diagnosis of MDD hinges on one or more principal symptoms, such as a depressed mood and anhedonia. The diagnostic standards for these symptoms are outlined in DSM-5-TR (American Psychiatric Association 2022) and ICD-10 (World Health Organization 1992). These two classification systems contain equivalent diagnostic criteria.

In research environments, diagnosing MDD adheres to a similar method. However, it leverages structured interviews that meticulously review MDD criteria while ruling out other psychiatric disorders through methodically structured questioning. Most research studies typically use the Mini-International Neuropsychiatric Interview (Sheehan et al. 1998) or the Structured Clinical Interview for DSM-5 Disorders—Clinician Version (First et al. 2016) as the primary diagnostic tool. Although comprehensive, these structured interviews can take 30–90 minutes to administer, often resulting in their exclusion from regular clinical practice.

It is crucial to note that the diagnosis of depression, as defined by these diagnostic standards, does not rest on any pathophysiological basis. No objective, quantifiable tests, such as blood tests, electroencephalograms (EEGs), or MRI scans, can confirm the diagnosis of depression or substantiate its presence. The diagnostic process, as it stands, relies entirely on subjective assessment without any corroborating biological evidence.

Treatment Phases for Major Depressive Disorder

Phases in the management of a depressive episode involve acute, continuation, and maintenance treatments. This perspective is important when using antidepressant pharmacotherapy and psychotherapy for initial or recurrent depressive episodes. The usual time frame for *acute treatment* is 6–12 weeks to achieve a response or remission of symptoms. Research shows that *continuation treatment* with pharmacotherapy and/or psychotherapy for an additional 4–12 months reduces the likelihood of relapse (e.g., Dobson et al. 2008). *Maintenance treatment* is the next step (i.e., beyond 4–12 months), and evidence supports the efficacy of such treatment protocols for recurrent forms of depression (e.g., Keller et al. 2007).

Experience indicates that recurrent forms of depression are more difficult to treat than an initial acute depressive episode. Furthermore, data from the largest real-world outcome trial (i.e., the Sequenced Treatment Alternatives to Relieve Depression [STAR*D] study) reported a decrease in the rate of antidepressant response with repeated treatment failures (Gaynes et al. 2009). For example, those who experience three failed treatment trials have a low (about 15%) rate of remission in a subsequent trial (see Table 2–1). These data are similar to the results of a 2-year study of treatment as usual for individuals who experienced multiple failed antidepressant treatments (Dunner et al. 2006).

Of note, the overall effect sizes (ESs) of antidepressants (ES=0.3), second-generation antipsychotics for augmentation (ES=0.26–0.48), and various psychotherapies (ES=0.22) indicate only modest clinical relevance (e.g., Cuijpers et al. 2009; Spielmans et al. 2013). Thus, these data should be carefully considered in one's risk-benefit assessment.

Those who do not respond to treatment with psychotherapy or antidepressant pharmacotherapy are considered to have *TRD* or *difficult-to-treat depression (DTD)*. The latter term takes into consideration continuing burden despite adequate treatment efforts due to difficulties

- Achieving and sustaining acute response or remission
- Addressing unacceptable tolerability and safety issues
- Returning to premorbid functionality and quality of life despite symptom control
- Accepting treatment options (McAllister-Williams et al. 2020)

Furthermore, sustained remission for patients with TRD or DTD is difficult to achieve with currently available options. A patient who attains remission after one prior antidepressant treatment failure has a 40% chance of relapse over the next year, whereas a patient who has attained remission after three prior antidepressant treatment failures has a 65% chance of relapse (Sackeim 2016; Warden et al. 2007).

Although studies indicate that electroconvulsive therapy (ECT) is the most effective acute antidepressant treatment for TRD or DTD in community settings, it is difficult to achieve sustained remission with this

Table 2–1. Acute-phase remission rates and continuation-phase relapse rates for patients with increasing treatment resistance

STAR*D level[a]	Acute-phase remission rate (%)	Continuation-phase relapse rate (%)
1	37	40
2	31	55
3	14	65
4	13	71

[a]Sequenced Treatment Alternatives to Relieve Depression (STAR*D) study levels: 1=initial treatment; 2=failure to remit with level 1 treatment; 3=failure to remit with level 2 treatment; 4=failure to remit with level 3 treatment (Warden et al. 2007).

modality. In a prospective, naturalistic study involving 347 patients at 7 hospitals, clinical outcomes immediately after ECT and over a 24-week follow-up period were examined in relation to patient characteristics and treatment variables (Prudic et al. 2004). Remission rates during the acute phase were documented in the range of 30%–45%, in contrast to the 70% rates observed in research studies. Likewise, the probability of relapse during the continuation phase was as high as 64%. Although patients who did not achieve remission during the acute phase had a poorer prognosis, the chance of relapse was high for all patients.

Neurocircuitry of Depression

MDD is a complex condition influenced by a mix of biological and environmental factors rather than a single cause. It is increasingly viewed as a *network disorder* characterized by altered activity within and between distinct functional networks. Critical networks include the default mode network, salience network, and central executive network (Bertocci et al. 2023). Specific connectivity abnormalities have been identified between the subgenual anterior cingulate cortex (sgACC), an integral node of the default mode network, and the dorsolateral prefrontal cortex (DLPFC), which is part of both the salience network and the central executive network. The DLPFC is thought to control sgACC activity from the top down, but this control is diminished in depression (Mayberg 2003).

The DLPFC, especially the left side, is the most common target for transcranial magnetic stimulation (TMS) treatment as a result of imaging studies showing decreased left prefrontal activity and increased right prefrontal activity (Grimm et al. 2008). Other potential targets implicated in depression's pathophysiology include the dorsomedial PFC, the ventro-medial PFC, the orbital frontal cortex, the parietal and temporal cortical areas, the ACC, parts of the striatum, the thalamus, and the hypothala-mus (see Figure 2–1). The DLPFC's superficial location makes it easily ac-cessible for TMS.

Although targeting the DLPFC with TMS to treat MDD is essential, it is important to note that depression is not caused merely by underactivity in the left prefrontal area or overactivity in the right prefrontal area. In-stead, the clinical effects of TMS depend on the transsynaptic propagation of signals throughout a distributed set of cortical and limbic regions.

Significant evidence suggests that the functional connectivity between DLPFC and sgACC may be critical to the response to TMS treatment in depression (Cash et al. 2019; Fox et al. 2012). Recent work suggested that these correlated and anticorrelated subregions are part of different affective circuits; stimulating a subregion of the left DLPFC that is anticorrelated with the sgACC reduces melancholic symptoms. In contrast, targeting a left DLPFC subregion correlated with the sgACC reduces anxious-somatic symptoms (Siddiqi et al. 2020). In this context, a growing body of evidence indicates that decreased activity in the left DLPFC and increased activity in the sgACC are the primary network dysfunctions in depression.

In this chapter, we review the efficacy of TMS on the basis of results from the key treatment studies for major depression. In this context, treat-ment parameters such as stimulus location, frequency, and intensity are also discussed.

General Overview of TMS Parameters

Clinical use of TMS is usually described in terms of four parameters:

1. *Location:* brain region stimulated
2. *Frequency:* pulses per second, intertrain interval, and frequency of treatment sessions
3. *Intensity:* expressed as a percentage of resting motor threshold (RMT)
4. *Duration:* pulses per treatment session and total number of treatment sessions

Together, these parameters determine the neurophysiological effects of TMS and form the basis for its dosage and administration. To treat de-pression, the two most important parameters are stimulus location (cor-tical target) and stimulus frequency. They are reviewed in detail. Other relevant parameters, such as the stimulus intensity, pulse number, pulse train interval, and number of treatment sessions, are briefly discussed.

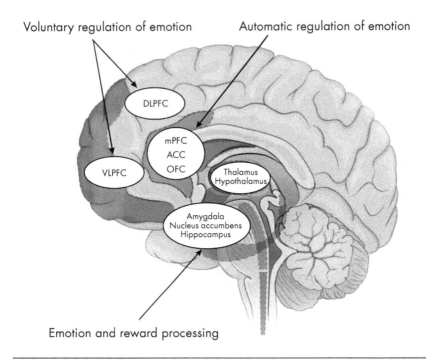

Figure 2-1. Depression circuit in the brain.

Left-sided lateral view of the brain, indicating the key structures and functions implicated in the pathophysiology of major depressive disorder:

Dorsolateral prefrontal cortex (DLPFC) and medial prefrontal cortex (mPFC)—executive function, regulation of emotion and assessment of consequences in decision-making, and extensive connections with anterior cingulate cortex (ACC) and limbic areas, including the hippocampus and amygdala;

Orbitofrontal cortex (OFC)—integration of multimodal stimuli and assessment of stimulus value and/or reward;

Ventrolateral prefrontal cortex (VLPFC)—attentional control;

ACC—extensive connections with brain structures implicated in emotional behavior, key part of an extended network in emotional processing and autonomic regulation;

Thalamus—sensory relay and extensive connections with limbic system and mood-related circuitry;

Hypothalamus—linking of the nervous system to the endocrine system and synthesizing and secreting of neurohormones, including corticotropin-releasing factor, a key structure in controlling hypothalamic-pituitary-adrenal (HPA) axis function;

Amygdala—evaluation of experience and stimuli with strong emotional valence and acquisition and expression of emotionally laden memories;

Nucleus accumbens—reward, pleasure, and pain avoidance; and

Hippocampus—learning, memory, cognition, site of adult neurogenesis, and negative regulation of the HPA axis.

Stimulus Location

The effects of TMS depend on which brain region is stimulated. For example, stimulating the motor cortex produces an immediately observable response in the form of a contralateral skeletal muscle contraction. Stimulating the occipital cortex can produce the subjective experience of flashing lights (phosphenes). Stimulating Broca's area can cause momentary speech arrest. Stimulating most other cortical areas, however, produces no immediate observable or subjective response. This is clearly the case with TMS treatment for depression, in that clinical results are typically seen only after several weeks of stimulation.

The most common stimulus target for TMS treatment of depression is the DLPFC, especially over the left side. The superficial location of the DLPFC is well within the TMS-induced electrical field, making it the most easily accessible target. Activating high-frequency (HF) protocols are typically applied over the left DLPFC, and inhibitory low-frequency (LF) protocols are typically applied over the right DLPFC.

Treatment Site Determination

Several methods are used to determine the stimulation site.

Five-Centimeter Rule

The 5-cm rule involves isolating the motor cortex area corresponding to the contralateral abductor pollicis brevis muscle and moving the coil 5 cm anteriorly. This method was used in the original pivotal trial leading to FDA clearance as well as in many early studies. The chief drawback of the 5-cm rule is that it fails to account for differences in head size and, in up to a third of patients, may miss the DLPFC target.

Neuronavigation

When neuronavigation is accessible, an individual's MRI can be aligned with a standard brain template, typically from the Montreal Neurological Institute (Evans et al. 1993). This procedure adjusts for variations in head size and shape. Subsequently, the stimulation site can be projected onto the scalp based on a Montreal Neurological Institute coordinate selected from a published study or an individualized imaging analysis.

However, incorporating MRI-guided coil placement into regular clinical practice is challenging because of various practical constraints, including additional costs, accessibility issues, and the complexity of most systems, which are often hard to operate and require substantial staff training. Consequently, MRI neuronavigation is seldom used in TMS clinics because the added implementation demands are not justified by the sporadic improvement in depression outcomes compared with more practical, easy-to-implement targeting methods (Fitzgerald et al. 2009; Li et al. 2020).

Another limitation of MRI-guided coil placement is that it does not target functionally connected brain areas. That is, it is based on structural rather than functional brain connectivity. This limitation is overcome using *functional* MRI–guided coil placement based on evidence that the degree of negative correlation, or anticorrelation, between the DLPFC stimulation site and the sgACC accounts for a large degree of the depression response or clinical efficacy of TMS (Cole et al. 2020; Siddiqi et al. 2019; Williams et al. 2018). Because of translational limitations, both structural and functional MRI–guided coil placements are rarely used outside academic research settings.

Electroencephalogram F3 Method

The EEG F3 method considers variations in head size and has accuracy similar to that of neuronavigation. This method relies on the International 10–20 System for EEG electrode placement, as described by Cardenas et al. (2022). In this method, the target is the F3 EEG site, which corresponds to the DLPFC. Normally, this is a derived location obtained only after first taking a series of painstaking measurements. William Beam at the Medical University of South Carolina, however, developed a streamlined method of locating F3 that requires only three simple measurements: tragus to tragus, nasion to inion, and head circumference (Beam et al. 2009). Entering these measurements into an equation yields a set of coordinates that can be easily marked on the patient's scalp, directly corresponding to F3 (see http://clinicalresearcher.org/eeg). This so-called Beam F3 method was compared with neuronavigation and found to be comparable to within 3 mm (Mir-Moghtadaei et al. 2015). Thus, it is now frequently used in routine clinical practice. Of note, the same measurement technique is easily modified to identify the F4 location on the right.

In a recent study involving a prospective, randomized, double-blind comparative effectiveness trial, researchers evaluated the clinical outcomes of the two different methods in a real-world group of patients with MDD who were undergoing TMS treatment. The results showed that the two DLPFC TMS targeting methods, Beam F3 and the 5.5-cm rule, produced comparable antidepressant effects (Trapp et al. 2023). These findings suggest that there is no significant difference in clinical outcomes for MDD patients with a head circumference of 60 cm or less, supporting the notion of clinical equipoise in this specific population.

Other Methods

Although valid at the group level, the 5-cm rule and Beam F3 method do not take into account individual variability. Functional and structural neuronavigation do take individual variability into account; however, they are time-consuming, expensive, and operationally difficult to implement. One emerging method for identifying a functionally meaningful site on the basis of the connectivity of the DLPFC to the sgACC involves the brain-heart connection (Iseger et al. 2017). Top-down modulation of heart rate by the PFC involves a frontal-vagal pathway from the PFC and anterior cingulate to subcortical nodes, including a monosynaptic pathway to the nucleus tractus solitarius of the vagus nerve. TMS applied to the PFC reduces heart rate by stimulation of this frontal-vagal network. This neuro-cardiac-guided TMS (NCG TMS) attempts to identify the most effective treatment site by determining the prefrontal area associated with the greatest degree of heart rate deceleration. This theory suggests that the effect on parasympathetic activity could be used as a functional outcome indicator to verify the appropriate targeting of the DLPFC-sgACC network. This is analogous to the way motor-evoked potential serves as a crucial functional measure for primary motor cortex stimulation. Specific subregions of the DLPFC appear to engage this circuit, and this method demonstrated sound test-retest reliability and a dose-response relationship between heart rate effects and stimulation intensity as defined by the percentage of maximum machine output (Iseger et al. 2021; Kaur et al. 2020). A further question that deserves attention is whether stimulation sites detected with the NCG TMS method will eventually lead to a superior clinical outcome in MDD.

Stimulus Frequency

High-Frequency TMS

The most common application of TMS for treating depression involves 10-Hz HF stimulation over the left DLPFC with a figure-eight coil. This method was used in the pivotal trials leading to FDA clearance of TMS in the United States (George et al. 2010; O'Reardon et al. 2007). In addition to these multicenter studies, numerous single-site studies demonstrated the efficacy of 10-Hz stimulation (e.g., Avery et al. 2008). However, substantial evidence also supports the use of up to 20-Hz stimulation. For example, the H1 coil stimulates at a frequency of 18 Hz. Although evidence suggests that multiple frequencies of 5 Hz or more have antidepressant effects, it is not clear which frequency is most beneficial for a given individual.

Low-Frequency TMS

A body of evidence also supports the efficacy of 1-Hz LF stimulation over the right DLPFC (e.g., Pallanti et al. 2010). A large sham-controlled study reported a response rate of 51% (Fitzgerald et al. 2006). Several direct comparison studies reported that LF TMS over the right DLPFC is as effective as HF TMS over the left DLPFC (e.g., Schutter 2010). In addition to comparable clinical efficacy, LF TMS is better tolerated by some patients, with fewer reports of pain or headache. It also may reduce the risk of seizure.

Combined High- and Low-Frequency TMS

HF and LF TMS are not mutually exclusive. These modalities may be administered in conjunction with each other in several ways (i.e., switching, sequential bilateral [SBL], and priming).

Switching refers to changing protocols because of a lack of response or lack of tolerability. For example, in one study of LF TMS, a subset of nonresponders subsequently responded when switched to HF TMS (Fitzgerald et al. 2006). Although these protocols may act through different mechanisms and some patient groups may be more responsive to specific protocols, it is also possible that the initial nonresponders would have responded if they had received a longer treatment course.

SBL treatment refers to the administration of both HF and LF TMS during the same treatment session. Although some clinicians believe that SBL treatment is superior in certain subgroups of patients (i.e., patients with high levels of anxiety), a meta-analysis of seven randomized controlled trials comparing unilateral and bilateral TMS ($N=509$) found no clear additional benefit with bilateral stimulation (Chen et al. 2014). Furthermore, results from a large repository of outcomes data (Aaronson et al. 2022) suggest that clinical outcomes of those who receive SBL treatment may, in fact, be inferior to those of patients who receive HF left unilateral treatment.

Priming stimulation is another option that involves the combination of HF and LF unilateral TMS. In this protocol, the application of several subthreshold HF trains (usually 6 Hz) is followed by standard LF stimulation over the right DLPFC (Iyer et al. 2003).

Although multiple TMS protocols are effective, evidence to date has not shown clear superiority of one protocol over another. A systematic review and network meta-analysis involving 81 studies ($N=4,233$) found few differences in clinical efficacy among left-sided HF stimulation, right-sided LF stimulation, and SBL stimulation (Brunoni et al. 2017).

Theta Burst Stimulation

Intermittent theta burst stimulation (iTBS) (see Chapter 1, "Basic Principles of Transcranial Magnetic Stimulation") applied to the left DLPFC, continuous theta burst stimulation (cTBS) applied to the right DLPFC, and SBL stimulation (i.e., iTBS and cTBS) are safe, well tolerated, and effective in treating depression (Voigt et al. 2021). One potential advantage to TBS protocols is that a treatment session is administered in 3–10 minutes compared with 20–45 minutes or more using most conventional TMS protocols. This increased efficiency could, at least in some circumstances, improve access and increase the availability of TMS. Additionally, because of the brevity of each session, TBS lends itself well to accelerated treatment protocols (i.e., protocols that involve two or more TMS sessions a day). For example, a sham-controlled trial reported significantly greater improvement in Montgomery-Åsberg Depression Rating Scale (MADRS) scores with active treatment using the Stanford Neuromodulation Therapy protocol (previously referred to as the Stanford Accelerated Intelligent Neuromodulation Therapy [SAINT] protocol). This is a high-dose, left-sided iTBS protocol using functional connectivity–guided targeting during 10 daily treatment sessions over 5 consecutive days (Cole et al. 2022).

Other TMS Parameters

Stimulus Intensity

Early TMS studies using stimulus intensities of 80%–90% of RMT generated mixed results. The FDA pivotal trial used a stimulus intensity of 120% RMT, which was virtually unprecedented at the time. As a result, it was proposed that suprathreshold stimulation is an important parameter in determining antidepressant efficacy. However, other parameters in this study were also different, including pulses per session and duration of treatment course. In fact, there are relatively few data regarding the efficacy of treatment based on stimulus intensity relative to RMT. Stimulus intensity does have implications for safety and tolerability, however, because higher intensity is associated with increased risk of posttreatment headache and seizure induction.

Motor threshold (MT) determination, coil placement, frequency choice, and other essential elements of correct TMS dosage are the responsibility of the treating clinician and should not be delegated to a technician or another assistant. These and other best practice guidelines are contained in the "Clinical TMS Society Consensus Review and Treatment Recommendations for TMS Therapy for Major Depressive Disorder" (Perera et al. 2016).

Pulse Trains and Pulses per Session

The original protocol cleared by the FDA specified an interval of 26 seconds between each 4-second train of 10-Hz stimulation delivered at 120% RMT. In 2017, a new protocol was FDA approved with a shorter interval of 11 seconds, thereby reducing a 38-minute treatment session to 19 minutes (Carpenter et al. 2021). In fact, many TMS practitioners were already using intervals as short as twice the length of the pulse train with no reported increase in the incidence of seizures or other adverse effects.

Early TMS studies involved the application of only several hundred pulses per session. The use of 3,000 pulses (75 pulse trains) in the FDA pivotal trials was considered novel and risky at the time but was surprisingly well tolerated and became the norm for most left-sided HF TMS protocols (Janicak et al. 2008). Increasing the pulse number in individual sessions, for example, to 5,000 pulses per session, in a pragmatic prospective trial did not substantially improve outcomes (Fitzgerald et al. 2020). However, in another large repository trial, patients who received more than 4,000 pulses per session of HF stimulation to the left DLPFC had superior outcomes (Sackeim et al. 2020).

Sessions per Treatment Course

The FDA pivotal trial involved a course of 30 treatments administered 5 days/week for 6 weeks followed by a 3-week tapering of the number of sessions per week. Thus, this 36-session treatment course became the norm and is covered by most U.S. insurance plans. Evidence indicates that increasing the total number of sessions per treatment course can improve outcomes or at least increase the total number of patients who respond (e.g., Avery et al. 2008).

Treatments are usually administered 5 days/week, but at least two studies reported that overall outcome is the same when treatments are administered 3 days/week in a course that is correspondingly longer (e.g., Galletly et al. 2012). No evidence suggests that administering treatment 7 days/week hastens recovery or produces a better outcome. One study suggested that the overall length of treatment may be shortened by administering multiple treatments over several days, without any increase in risk (Holtzheimer et al. 2010). Another study found that three TMS treatments per day over the course of 3 days brought about a rapid decrease in suicidal ideation (George et al. 2014).

Most patients adapt quickly to the stimulus sensation, and premature discontinuation of treatment is uncommon. The structure provided by daily treatments and the interpersonal contact as part of the session may provide therapeutic value for some patients and are worthy of further study.

Improvement occurs gradually and is like the time course seen with antidepressant medication. Most patients notice improvement between 15 and 20 treatments, although earlier and later responses may occur. Core somatic symptoms (e.g., sleep, appetite, and energy) typically improve before subjective sadness and other psychological symptoms, and family or friends may notice changes first. Interestingly, many patients report a change in visual perception (e.g., colors appear more vivid), along with improved clarity of thinking and improved memory.

Regular follow-up is essential. Standardized rating scales such as the 9-item Personal Health Questionnaire (PHQ-9) and Quick Inventory of Depressive Symptomatology provide quantifiable measures of symptom severity. Furthermore, their use is routinely required by many insurance plans to justify the ongoing need for treatment.

Acute Efficacy of TMS Treatment for Treatment-Resistant Depression

Pivotal Depression Study

FDA clearance of TMS was based on a precise treatment protocol delivered by a specific device in a large ($N=301$) multisite ($N=23$) randomized sham-controlled trial (O'Reardon et al. 2007). Patients in this study did not respond to at least one and no more than four adequate antidepressant medication trials and, except for limited use of sedative-anxiolytics, were medication free at the time of the study.

When this pivotal trial was designed, it was not clear how long patients needed to be treated. Many previous studies lasted only 2 weeks, much less than the time usually required for medications (6–8 weeks) or ECT (2–4 weeks) to take effect. Also unclear were the overall intensity of stimulation and number of pulses required.

In the pivotal study, treatment was provided 5 days/week (Monday through Friday) for 4–6 weeks, followed by a 3-week tapering phase. Thus, patients could receive up to 36 sessions of TMS therapy over 9 weeks. The treatment protocol used high-intensity, HF stimulation of 10 Hz at 120% of MT delivered over the left DLPFC. Each treatment session involved seventy-five 4-second-long pulse trains interspersed by a

26-second intertrain interval, totaling 3,000 pulses. This duration and this intensity of stimulation were unprecedented at the time.

Active TMS was significantly superior to sham TMS on the basis of change from the baseline scores on the MADRS at week 4 (with a post hoc correction for inequality in symptom severity between groups at baseline). Furthermore, results were similar on the secondary outcome measures (i.e., 17- and 24-item Hamilton Depression Rating Scale [HDRS-17 and -24] at weeks 4 and 6). Response rates were also significantly higher with active TMS than with sham TMS on all three scales at weeks 4 and 6. Remission rates were approximately twofold higher with active TMS than with sham TMS at week 6 and were significantly higher on the MADRS and HDRS-24 (but not the HDRS-17). Active TMS produced adverse effects that were generally mild, and most involved transient scalp discomfort or pain, with an associated low dropout rate (4.5%) (Janicak et al. 2008; O'Reardon et al. 2007).

Patients who did not achieve a predetermined improvement level of benefit from at least 4 weeks of randomized treatment assignment in the controlled trial (either active or sham) were eligible to participate in an open-label extension trial. Of note, patients and investigators remained blind to prior assignment at the time of entry into this phase (Avery et al. 2008). For those patients who received sham TMS in the initial randomized controlled trial ($N=85$), the mean reduction in MADRS scores after 6 weeks of open-label active TMS was 17.0. Furthermore, on the basis of the MADRS score reduction at 6 weeks, 36 of these patients (42.4%) achieved response, and 17 patients (20.0%) achieved remission (i.e., MADRS score <10). For those patients who received but did not respond to active TMS in the initial randomized controlled trial ($N=73$), the mean reduction in MADRS scores was 12.5, and response and remission rates were 26.0% and 11.0%, respectively. This finding seems to indicate that a substantial number of patients require a longer than average course of TMS.

Optimization of TMS for Depression Study

An independent (non-industry-sponsored) National Institute of Mental Health–sponsored study, Optimization of TMS for Depression (OPT-TMS), used the same device and same treatment parameters as the pivotal study but also included some methodological improvements. Thus, it included MRI adjustment for coil placement, an adaptive flexible duration of treatment, an improved sham device that better mimicked the sensory experience of TMS, and continuous assessment of outcome evaluator reliability relative to a masked external expert rater (George et al. 2010). High-intensity TMS for at least 3 weeks was significantly more likely than sham TMS to induce remission (the primary end point in this trial) in patients with moderately treatment-resistant unipolar MDD who were not taking antidepressant medication. The level of treatment resistance in this study was higher than in the FDA pivotal registration study.

The H1 TMS Depression Study

Hesed or H coils have been put forward as a method to efficiently stimulate deeper brain structures. Because of their intricate windings and larger size in comparison with standard figure-eight coils, H coils are projected to exhibit a slower rate of electrical field decay with increasing depth, albeit with diminished focality. The H coil induces cortical excitability up to a maximum depth of 4–5 cm, whereas figure-eight coils penetrate to a depth of 1.5–3 cm (Deng et al. 2013). Therefore, it is able to directly modulate the activity of both the cerebral cortex and deeper neural circuits (Bersani et al. 2013).

The FDA cleared the BrainsWay Deep TMS System H1 coil in 2013. This approval was based on a study involving an intent-to-treat sample of 212 patients at 20 sites in 4 different countries. All patients had previously not responded to as many as four adequate antidepressant medication trials during the current episode and were randomly assigned to receive either active deep TMS or sham treatment. Patients, treaters, and raters were fully blinded. A total of 181 patients completed the study per protocol. Acute treatment consisted of five sessions per week for 4 weeks, followed by a continuation phase of twice-weekly treatment for 12 more weeks. The stimulation site was the left DLPFC, although broader stimulation was likely with the H1 coil. Stimulation parameters were 120% of MT, frequency of 18 Hz, train duration of 2 seconds, intertrain interval of 20 seconds, and 55 trains per session, for a total of 1,980 pulses over 20 minutes (Levkovitz et al. 2015).

The primary end point in this study was the change in total score on the 21-item HDRS (HDRS-21) from baseline to week 5. The secondary efficacy end points were response and remission rates at week 5. Response was defined as a reduction of at least 50% in the total HDRS-21 score compared with baseline, and remission was defined as a total HDRS-21 score lower than 10.

In the intent-to-treat sample, the difference of –2.23 points (95% CI= –4.54, 0.07) between the slopes across 5 weeks fell just short of reaching statistical significance (P=0.058). However, the study results were analyzed for a subset of patients who received the prescribed stimulation protocol at 120% of MT (n=181, 89 in the TMS sample and 92 in the sham sample). In this subsample of patients, the difference of –3.11 points

(95% CI=−5.40, −0.83) between the slopes was statistically significant ($P=0.008$), with an effect size of 0.76.

In terms of the secondary outcome measures, at week 5, the response rates (prescribed stimulation protocol set) were 38.4% for active treatment versus 21.4% for sham TMS ($P=0.014$), and remission rates (prescribed stimulation protocol set) were 32.6% for active treatment versus 14.6% for sham TMS. At week 16, the response rates were 44.3% for active treatment versus 25.6% for sham TMS, and remission rates were 31.8% for active treatment versus 22.2% for sham TMS.

To date, very few studies have compared H1-coil TMS with standard figure-eight-coil TMS. However, Filipčić et al. (2019) conducted a single-center, three-arm, randomized controlled trial to assess the outcomes of two FDA-approved repetitive TMS protocols—H1 coil and figure-eight coil—in patients with MDD. A total of 228 patients were randomly assigned to receive 20 sessions of either H1-coil or figure-eight-coil TMS, both as adjuncts to standard pharmacotherapy, or standard pharmacotherapy alone. The study found significantly higher remission rates in the high-frequency repetitive TMS groups compared with the control group. However, no significant difference in remission rates was observed between the H1-coil and the figure-eight-coil groups. The H1-coil group had better response rates and greater reductions in depression severity than the figure-eight-coil group. Both repetitive TMS modalities were equally safe and well tolerated.

Similarly, Gellersen and Kedzior (2019) systematically compared the antidepressant effects of figure-eight-coil repetitive TMS and deep TMS with those of the H1 coil in studies matched for stimulation frequency in unipolar MDD. Their analysis suggested that, at the same frequency, the H1 coil's higher-intensity, less-focal stimulation was more effective in reducing depression than the figure-eight coil's lower-intensity, more-focal approach.

Theta Burst Stimulation Depression Studies

In another trial, a TMS protocol using iTBS demonstrated benefit comparable to that of standard TMS without greater risks. It was a large ($N=385$) randomized noninferiority study in patients with TRD who received iTBS TMS. As noted earlier in the "Theta Burst Stimulation" subsection, iTBS TMS allows for an accelerated session time (i.e., ~3.5 vs. ~37.5 minutes/session) (Blumberger et al. 2018). The clinical relevance is the substantial reduction in the time commitment per treatment session.

The same group conducted a second open, randomized noninferiority trial ($N=172$) using blinded raters to ascertain the effectiveness and tolerability of bilateral TBS compared with standard bilateral TMS in *older adults* (age >60 years) with TRD. They reported reductions in depression symptoms, low all-cause dropout rates, and comparable tolerability (including cognitive measures) within the two groups (Blumberger et al. 2022). Although the trial was designed as a noninferiority trial, the TBS arm performed better than standard bilateral TMS on all measures and outcomes. The TBS arm showed an ongoing improvement up to 4 weeks posttreatment that was superior to standard TMS. This finding of sustained and progressive improvement is consistent with the possibility that TBS induces greater brain plasticity than standard TMS protocols (Di Lazzaro et al. 2011). The substantial reduction in session time in the TBS group (4 minutes) compared with bilateral TMS (48 minutes) may provide significant clinical benefit and more access to patients with TRD. Table 2–2 summarizes the results of the five large pivotal trials.

Effectiveness in Real-World Patients

In addition to the studies described in the "Theta Burst Stimulation Depression Studies" subsection, several multisite, naturalistic observational studies examined the safety and long-term effectiveness of TMS in clinical populations. These studies are important because they more accurately reflect the administration of TMS in a real-world setting. For example, both the FDA pivotal study and the OPT-TMS study excluded patients with disorders other than major depression (except for simple phobia and nicotine addiction). In typical clinical practice, however, many patients receiving TMS have comorbid psychiatric illness such as an eating disorder or PTSD or a history of psychosis. Similarly, in both the FDA pivotal registration study and the OPT-TMS study, patients were required to be medication free for 1 week prior to the start of the study. That is almost never the case in the real world, where virtually all patients with depression are taking one or more psychotropic medications, often from different classes.

Carpenter et al. (2012) examined outcomes in 307 patients treated at 42 clinical TMS practice sites in the United States. Most received the standard FDA-cleared protocol associated with the Neuronetics device (see Figure 9–3 in Chapter 9, "Current FDA-Cleared Transcranial Magnetic Stimulation Systems"). The clinician-assessed response rate based on the Clinical Global Impression—Severity of Illness Scale (CGI-S) was 58.0%, and the remission rate was 37.1%. Patient-reported response rates ranged from 56.4% to 41.5%, and remission rates ranged from 28.7% to 26.5% on the basis of the PHQ-9 and Inventory of Depressive Symptomatology—Self-Report, respectively. Overall, these outcomes were similar to those seen in research populations.

Table 2–2. Key studies demonstrating TMS efficacy in major depressive disorder

Type of study	rTMS	Sample	Response rate (%)	Remission rate (%)	Comments
Randomized controlled, multisite, blinded trial (O'Reardon et al. 2007)	75 trains per day of 10-Hz stimulation (3,000 pulses)	301 patients with TRD	23.9 (active) vs. 15.1 (sham)	17.4 (active) vs. 8.2 (sham)	Figure-eight coil, subjects were medication free, remission and response rates at 6 weeks
Randomized controlled, multisite, blinded trial (George et al. 2010)	75 trains per day of 10-Hz stimulation (3,000 pulses)	190 patients with TRD	15 (active) vs. 5 (sham)	14.1 (active) vs. 5.1 (sham)	Figure-eight coil, subjects were medication free, remission and response rates at 3 weeks
Randomized controlled, multisite, blinded trial (Levkovitz et al. 2015)	55 trains per day of 20-Hz stimulation (1,980 pulses), deep TMS coil	212 patients with TRD, 181 patients in per-protocol analysis	38.4 (active) vs. 21.4 (sham)	32.6 (active) vs. 14.5 (sham)	H1 coil, subjects were medication free, remission and response rates at 5 weeks

Table 2–2. Key studies demonstrating TMS efficacy in major depressive disorder *(continued)*

Type of study	rTMS	Sample	Response rate (%)	Remission rate (%)	Comments
Randomized controlled, noninferiority trial, blinded raters (Blumberger et al. 2018)	TMS: 75 trains per day of 10-Hz stimulation (3,000 pulses) iTBS: 600 pulses over 189 seconds	385 patients with TRD	47 (TMS) vs. 49 (iTBS)	27 (TMS) vs. 32 (iTBS)	Figure-eight coil, subjects were taking stable medication, remission and response rates at 4 weeks
Randomized controlled, noninferiority trial, blinded raters (Blumberger et al. 2022)	Standard sequential bilateral TMS: 1-Hz stimulation, 120% RMT, 600 pulses over 10 minutes to the right DLPFC, followed by 10-Hz stimulation, 120% RMT, 3,000 pulses for 4 seconds on, 26 seconds off, over 37.5 minutes to the left DLPFC compared with Sequential bilateral TBS: 120% RMT with right-sided cTBS, triplet burst pulses at 50 Hz, repeated at 5 Hz for 600 pulses over 40 seconds,	172 older adults with TRD; 87 participants received standard sequential bilateral TMS, and 85 received sequential TBS	44.3 (TBS) vs. 32.9 (TMS)	35.4 (TBS) vs. 32.9 (TMS)	Figure-eight coil, subjects were taking stable medication, remission and response rates at 4 weeks

Table 2–2. Key studies demonstrating TMS efficacy in major depressive disorder *(continued)*

Type of study	rTMS	Sample	Response rate (%)	Remission rate (%)	Comments
Randomized controlled, noninferiority trial, blinded raters (Blumberger et al. 2022) *(continued)*	followed by left-sided iTBS, triplet burst pulses at 50 Hz, repeated at 5 Hz, 2 seconds on, 8 seconds off, for 600 pulses over 3 minutes 9 seconds				

Note. cTBS=continuous TBS; DLPFC=dorsolateral prefrontal cortex; iTBS=intermittent TBS; RMT=resting motor threshold; rTMS=repetitive TMS; TBS=theta burst stimulation; TMS=transcranial magnetic stimulation; TRD=treatment-resistant depression.

To consider real-world outcomes of acute TMS treatment, Sackeim et al. (2020) analyzed data from patients with MDD in the NeuroStar Advanced Therapy System Clinical Outcomes Registry (N = 5,010 in the intention-to-treat sample; 103 practice sites). Approaches to delivering TMS included multiple protocols (i.e., HF left DLPFC, LF right DLPFC, and bilateral TMS). Overall, response and remission rates after more than 20 sessions were 58% and 28%, respectively.

Tendler et al. (2023) conducted an extensive postmarketing data analysis involving 1,753 patients from 21 different sites to examine real-world outcomes associated with acute deep TMS treatment. The authors found that response and remission rates after more than 20 sessions with this coil were 76% and 58%, respectively. Although these response and remission rates were higher than in the FDA registration trial and OPT-TMS study, the study populations and the primary outcome measures were different.

Systematic Reviews and Meta-Analyses of Acute TMS Studies

Summary evidence for the acute efficacy of TMS in TRD now includes more than 50 sham-controlled clinical studies involving more than 3,200 patients (Wang et al. 2022). Results from these trials were reported in multiple systematic reviews and meta-analyses and provide a consistent, comprehensive, and replicated literature base.

For example, Schutter (2009) evaluated 30 double-blind, sham-controlled studies involving 1,164 patients and found that HF TMS over the left DLPFC was superior to sham TMS, with an effect size comparable to that of commercially available antidepressant medications. In a larger study, Slotema et al. (2010) examined 34 sham-controlled studies involving 1,383 patients; they concluded that TMS is effective in treating depression and has a mild side-effect profile. In another meta-analysis, Gaynes et al. (2014) concluded that TMS is a reasonable and effective consideration for patients with major depression who experienced at least two previous antidepressant treatment failures and that patients receiving TMS were at least five times as likely to achieve remission as patients receiving sham TMS.

In their systematic review and meta-analysis, Sonmez et al. (2019) found that accelerated TMS protocols (e.g., increased number of stimulations per session and increased number of sessions per day) are effective and safe. In another systematic review and meta-analysis, Voigt et al. (2021) found that delivering TMS with TBS was superior to a sham procedure and noninferior to standard HF left DLPFC TMS.

Other Symptom Improvements in Major Depressive Disorder With TMS

Anxious Depression

Comorbid anxiety with MDD is common, and these conditions may have the same underlying pathophysiology. Hutton et al. (2023) assessed the potential role of TMS to manage anxiety in the context of MDD. They used data from the NeuroStar Advanced Therapy System Clinical Outcomes Registry to identify patients who met criteria for anxious depression (i.e., baseline Generalized Anxiety Disorder 7-item scale [GAD-7] score of 10 or greater; $N=1,514$). These patients reported clinically meaningful anxiolytic and antidepressant effects (i.e., 50% or greater reductions in both GAD-7 and PHQ-9 scores) following TMS. Among those with anxious depression, the change in anxiety and depression symptoms strongly covaried. Pell et al. (2022) similarly found that TMS with the H1 coil for MDD treatment was effective for both depressive and anxiety symptoms. Furthermore, higher baseline anxiety was found to be predictive of a successful outcome with the H1 coil treatment. These data were submitted to the FDA, and the BrainsWay Deep TMS System with the H1 coil received the FDA clearance for MDD with comorbid anxiety [510(k) No. K210201; www.accessdata.fda.gov/cdrh_docs/pdf21/K210201.pdf].

Suicidal Ideation

Weissman et al. (2018) pooled data from two prospective randomized controlled trials of TMS over the DLPFC (bilateral, left unilateral, sham) for TRD ($N=156$). They focused on the suicide item of the HDRS-17 and reported that bilateral TMS was superior to sham TMS in reducing suicidal ideation. Notably, only a small portion of the reduction in suicidal ideation was attributable to the reduction in depressive symptoms. The investigators posited that suicidal ideation may be targeted with TMS.

In a second report, Mehta et al. (2022) pooled data from the Blumberger et al. (2018) randomized controlled trial that compared 10-Hz TMS and iTBS TMS given over the left DLPFC for TRD ($N=301$). They also focused on the suicide item of the HDRS-17 and reported that both 10-Hz TMS and iTBS TMS effectively reduced suicidality to a clinically meaningful degree. Of note, patients with more severe suicidal ideation were excluded from this trial.

Quality of Life

Functional status and quality-of-life outcomes were assessed in 307 participants from the pivotal trial (Janicak et al. 2013; O'Reardon et al.

2007). Following acute TMS treatment, statistically significant improvement was observed in functional status in a broad range of mental health and physical health domains on the basis of the Medical Outcomes Study 36-item Short-Form Health Survey (SF-36). Similarly, statistically significant improvement in patient-reported quality of life was observed in all domains of the EuroQol 5-Dimensions questionnaire and in the General Health Perception and Health Index subscale scores. Improvement in these measures was observed across the entire range of baseline depression symptom severity, demonstrating that TMS as administered in routine clinical practice settings produces statistically and clinically meaningful improvements in patient-reported quality of life and functional status.

In a secondary analysis of data ($N=385$), Blumberger et al. (2018) assessed short- and long-term changes in self-reported quality of life (Quality of Life Enjoyment and Satisfaction Questionnaire) and disability (Sheehan Disability Scale) following 6 weeks of TMS. Changes in pretreatment scores at 1 week (acute follow-up) and at 12 weeks post treatment (long-term follow-up) were assessed. Scores improved significantly, with no differences in patient-reported outcomes between the treatment arms, either acutely or long term. Furthermore, the effect sizes were significantly greater in those who achieved better resolution of their depressive symptoms.

Cognition

Cognitive dysfunction is common in patients with MDD, often impairing activities such as attention, memory, and executive function. In this context, a systematic review of the literature was conducted to investigate the role of TMS in improving neurocognition in patients with TRD (Serafini et al. 2015). Twenty-two studies met the authors' inclusion criteria, with most suggesting a trend toward improvements in neurocognition with TMS. Although a few studies reported negative findings, either their interpretation was limited by small sample sizes or they included mixed samples or used single-blind designs, potentially compromising the study design.

Tapering Phase

TMS, similar to antidepressants, should be tapered rather than ended abruptly. Typically, a course of treatment will consist of approximately 25–30 treatments administered 5 days/week, followed by a tapering phase of 3 treatments for 1 week, 2 treatments the next week, and 1 treatment the final week as per the pivotal registration trial (O'Reardon et al. 2007).

Durability of Response After Acute TMS Treatment

Once a patient responds to TMS, how long will the benefit last? Most patients pose this question during the consent process because they have experienced the disappointment of initially benefiting from previous antidepressant treatments only to have their symptoms recur in the ensuing months.

The durability of TMS effect following acute treatment was established in several studies both with and without maintenance antidepressant medication. In general, these studies reported high durability for acute TMS benefits.

To investigate the mean remission time and the predictors associated with the treatment's duration, Cohen et al. (2009) performed a large retrospective, naturalistic study with 204 patients who underwent TMS therapy. Patients were followed up for up to 6 months after acute treatment, and about 80% took psychotropic medications. The rate of event-free remission, with the end point defined as relapse (i.e., HDRS scores >8), was 75.3% at 2 months, 60.0% at 3 months, 42.7% at 4 months, and 22.6% at 6 months. In summary, the mean duration of remission was approximately 4 months (119 days), with younger age and greater number of TMS sessions predicting greater durability of benefit.

Janicak et al. (2010) studied the durability of TMS in a population of 99 patients with MDD who had at least partially responded to acute TMS treatment while medication free. The patients then received antidepressant monotherapy for 24 weeks. If patients met predefined criteria for symptom worsening, they could receive TMS reintroduction (i.e., two sessions/week for 2 weeks and, if needed, five sessions/week for 4 additional weeks). Thirty-eight patients (38%) had symptom worsening and received TMS reintroduction. Of the 38 patients, 32 (84%) benefited, with the mean time to reintroduction of TMS being 109 days and the mean number of TMS reintroduction sessions being 14.3. Fifteen patients needed more than one course of TMS, and five patients needed up to three courses. Ten patients relapsed despite access to flexible reintroduction of TMS. In summary, TMS response was durable when patients were allowed to receive flexible reintroduction of TMS combined with antidepressant monotherapy.

Dunner et al. (2014) reported the 1-year outcome in 257 patients with MDD treated with TMS. The acute treatment response was reported by Carpenter et al. (2012). Because it was an observational study conducted across 42 clinical practices in the United States, all patients were permitted clinician-directed treatment as usual (i.e., patients were not limited to a predefined single antidepressant as in the Janicak et al. [2010] study). Most were given antidepressant medications, and many received other medications (e.g., second-generation antipsychotic augmentation) during the acute and follow-up periods. Patients were allowed TMS reintroduction after acute treatment if it was deemed appropriate and prescribed by their physician. Other treatments, such as psychotherapy, were not reported. Ninety-three patients were treated with TMS during the ensuing 12 months of follow-up; the mean number of TMS sessions for this group was 16.2. Of the 45 subjects who did not maintain their remission or response status, 31 relapsed within 6 months. In summary, more than 60% of the patients who had responded to or achieved remission during acute treatment with TMS sustained their response for 1 year. No safety or tolerability issues were noted during reintroduction of TMS.

Overall, these studies indicate that acute TMS therapy is beneficial for most patients with more chronic forms of depression for up to 12 months. Although research studies of TMS involved antidepressant medication–free patients, patients in these trials were transitioned to antidepressant monotherapy during the tapering phase of TMS. In clinical practice, most patients continue taking medication after TMS. Having access to flexible doses of TMS to treat recurrent symptoms during the continuation phase improves durability, and most patients with such access require fewer TMS sessions to maintain their remission or response status. Continuing medication and reintroducing TMS are effective, but more research is needed to determine the optimal strategy for keeping patients well. Randomized head-to-head studies comparing different protocols are needed.

Following TMS treatment, patients should be closely monitored, and their symptoms should be measured with a validated depression questionnaire. Research is needed to try to determine which patients are at the highest risk for relapse. Perhaps certain clinical or demographic variables predict relapse after TMS therapy. Several candidate variables were examined in the studies described in this section, but the results were inconsistent. Patients who achieve remission with acute TMS have the best prognosis for maintaining response.

Preventing Relapse or Recurrence After Acute Response to TMS

Because maintenance antidepressants and psychotherapy are effective in delaying a relapse or recurrence of depression, it would seem logical that providing TMS in some ongoing manner (*preservation TMS*) after response also would provide protection against relapse or recurrence (Wilson et al. 2022). Table 2–3 summarizes several published TMS maintenance studies. Before 2015, these studies were observational (retrospective or prospective) in design without a comparison group or involved case reports (e.g., Chatterjee et al. 2012; Demirtas-Tatlidede et al. 2008). Most defined *maintenance TMS* as scheduled sessions delivered weekly (e.g., one to two per week) with a taper to a frequency of once monthly delivered during the continuation phase. TMS delivered in this fashion preserved the response and remission rates obtained in the acute phase of treatment or at least delayed the decrement in the antidepressant effect achieved after the acute phase.

Two studies indicated that continuing TMS treatments after the acute series can prevent relapse or recurrence and can also improve remission and response rates. Harel et al. (2014) treated patients in three distinct phases: 1) an acute phase for 4 weeks, in which daily TMS sessions were conducted five times per week, for a total of 20 sessions; 2) a continuation treatment phase for 8 weeks, in which TMS sessions were conducted twice a week, for a total of 16 sessions; and 3) a second continuation treatment phase for 10 weeks, during which TMS sessions were conducted once a week. Patients also continued their antidepressant medications. A significant decrease in HDRS score from baseline was found at the end of the acute phase ($P < 0.001$) and was maintained throughout the 18-week study. Furthermore, the probability of response and remission increased over the course of the study, almost doubling for those who received continuation treatment.

Levkovitz et al. (2015) also included a continuation treatment phase. The investigators randomly assigned 212 patients with TRD to monotherapy with TMS or sham TMS. Patients received daily sessions for 4 weeks, and 159 patients were available to continue twice-weekly sessions for 18 weeks. Response and remission rates were higher in the TMS group than in the sham group ($P = 0.01$ response; $P = 0.005$ remission), and these benefits were preserved during the next 3 months with maintenance TMS.

Two reviews and a meta-analysis indicated that the benefits from TMS are preserved with scheduled TMS sessions or with monitoring and then reintroducing TMS when the symptoms recur. A systematic review of 19 studies published between 2002 and 2018 found that among initial responders, 66.5% sustained response at 3 months, 52.9% sustained response at 6 months, and 46.3% sustained response at 12 months (Senova et al. 2019). Random-effects meta-regressions demonstrated that receipt of maintenance of any form predicted higher responder rates at the spec-

Table 2–3. Maintenance studies of transcranial magnetic stimulation (TMS) for major depressive disorder

Study	Sample (N)	Design	Duration	Frequency of TMS	Outcome
O'Reardon et al. 2005	10	Retrospective	6 months to 6 years	1–2 sessions/week	3 patients maintained response
Connolly et al. 2012	42	Retrospective	6 months	Tapered to 1 session/month	62% maintained response
Fitzgerald et al. 2013	35	Prospective	1 year	5 clustered treatments over 2 days monthly	Delay in relapse
Richieri et al. 2013	59	Prospective	20 weeks	Tapered to 1 session/month	38% relapsed with maintenance, whereas 68% relapsed without maintenance
Harel et al. 2014	26	Prospective	18 weeks	Twice-weekly sessions for 8 weeks, then weekly	50% remission rate at end of study
Levkovitz et al. 2015	159	Prospective, sham controlled	12 weeks	Twice-weekly sessions	Active treatment superior to sham
Philip et al. 2016	49	Prospective, randomized	1 year	Monthly session	No significant differences between groups
Benadhira et al. 2017	17	Prospective, randomized, sham controlled	6 months	Month 1: 3 sessions/week for 2 weeks, 2 sessions/week for 2 weeks; Months 2–4: 1 session/week; Months 5–6: 1 session every other week	Active treatment superior to sham for months 1–4

ified time points. In another systematic review of TMS after the induction course, including continuation, maintenance, and rescue TMS, data were abstracted from 30 sources ($N=1,494$), including 4 randomized controlled trials (1 sham controlled), 14 open trials, and 12 cases series (Wilson et al. 2022). This research found that the quality of the existing literature is low regarding efficacy, but there is clear support for safety and effectiveness across a wide range of different TMS protocols to preserve patients' benefits after the acute course.

Given the various protocols to preserve patients' status after the induction course, it is difficult to know how to proceed clinically when patients are finishing their first acute course. In a pilot study, Philip et al. (2016) attempted to address this issue by comparing outcomes in patients who received either scheduled TMS or observation after a 6-week course of TMS therapy. Forty-nine patients who met response criteria at the end of the acute phase were randomly assigned to one treatment monthly or a monthly visit without TMS treatment during 12 months of follow-up. Patients in both groups who relapsed could receive reintroduction TMS. Importantly, patients remained medication free during the acute and follow-up periods. More than 80% of the patients in both groups met the criteria for remission at the end of acute treatment, defined as a score of 7 or less on the HDRS-17. Subsequently, no between-group difference was found in the number of patients who did not require TMS reintroduction (the primary outcome variable). However, TMS-treated patients had a slightly longer duration to first relapse (91 vs. 77 days), were slightly less likely to require retreatment with TMS (35% vs. 39%), required fewer retreatments in the case of relapse (14.3 vs. 16.9), and showed a slightly higher percentage of response to retreatment (78% vs. 63%). In summary, in this pilot study ($N=49$), the two approaches were comparable on the basis of the primary and secondary outcome measures.

In clinical practice, we recommend monitoring patients closely during the first 6 months after the first induction course. Monitoring should involve a combination of clinical assessments with validated instruments that are sensitive to changes in depressive symptoms. If a patient shows symptoms of recurrence, it is best to reintroduce TMS early rather than wait for full relapse criteria to be met. Reintroduction can be flexible, for example, two to three times a week for 2–3 weeks with a reduction in services based on the patient's response. For patients who require more than two TMS courses a year or who relapse frequently, we recommend scheduled TMS sessions with monthly assessments.

TMS has a durable antidepressant effect for patients with TRD or DTD when used as an adjunct to medication or monotherapy. Durability is en-

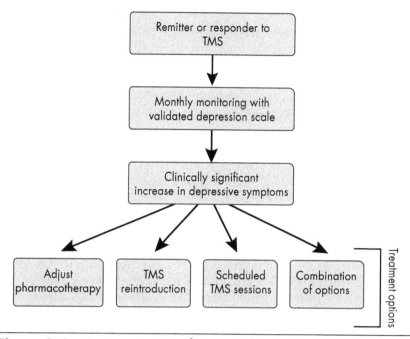

Figure 2–2. Treatment options for responders and remitters to optimize the durability of transcranial magnetic stimulation (TMS).

hanced when other treatments or reintroduction TMS is used during the continuation phase. The best way to optimize the durability of TMS remains unclear. Regardless of the coil design, stimulation site, or stimulation protocol, closely monitoring patients and reintroducing TMS early when symptoms emerge are the current standards of care.

Figure 2–2 provides several options for patients that may improve the durability of response or remission. Prescribers should consider a patient-centered approach that considers the individual's history of treatment response, the number and severity of depressive episodes, and the availability of continued TMS treatments because insurance coverage can greatly vary. Patients with TRD who respond to TMS should be managed with a combination of pharmacotherapy, psychotherapy, and TMS, with the goal of increasing the number of days spent in remission.

Conclusion

TMS represents a major advance in noninvasive therapeutic neuromodulation with proven efficacy in the treatment of MDD. Its safety and benign side-effect profile make it a viable treatment alternative for patients who do not respond to or tolerate antidepressant medication. TMS is a viable option to augment medication and has shown efficacy as a monotherapy. However, TMS is not a cure for MDD, and patients should be monitored closely for symptoms of depression after completing a course of TMS. Furthermore, TMS is best prescribed within the context of a biopsychosocial treatment plan and incorporated with psychotherapy and medication management for MDD. Modifications of TMS technique and improvements in TMS technology, including the development of new stimulation coils, may further enhance clinical efficacy (see Chapter 10, "Transcranial Magnetic Stimulation: Recent and Future Innovations").

Although the mechanism of action of TMS is not fully understood, evidence suggests that its therapeutic effects result from neuroplastic changes in thalamocortical circuits involved in the expression of core symptoms of major depression. Furthermore, the most effective stimulation sites appear to be individual targets within the PFC that show stronger functional anticorrelations with the sgACC (Fox et al. 2013). These findings, together with those derived from other lines of research, such as functional neuroimaging and brain lesion studies, shed light on the pathophysiology and circuit dysfunction associated with MDD.

KEY POINTS

- Transcranial magnetic stimulation (TMS) is an effective treatment for those who do not respond to antidepressant medication or psychotherapy, with benefits persisting for at least 1 year in some patients.

- The most common protocol for treating depression is as follows: stimulating the left dorsolateral prefrontal cortex with stimulus intensity at 120% of motor threshold and frequency at 10 Hz for 30–35 daily treatment sessions, Monday through Friday, each lasting ~5–37.5 minutes.

- Clinical improvement may be seen in 2–3 weeks but typically requires 30 or more treatments over 4–6 weeks.

- For patients who have partial improvement or response in 30 sessions, there is an added benefit to extending the acute course of TMS to obtain remission.

- Alternative TMS treatment protocols, such as theta burst stimulation, can substantially shorten treatment sessions and possibly accelerate the time to achieve benefit without increasing risk. Recent trials indicate that theta burst stimulation is not inferior to TMS; tolerability and safety are equivalent.

- Patients should have their moods assessed with a validated instrument (e.g., the 9-item Personal Health Questionnaire) at regular intervals for early identification of symptom recurrence because flexible access to TMS for symptom recurrence is an effective strategy to help patients maintain acute benefits.

References

Aaronson ST, Carpenter LL, Hutton TM, et al: Comparison of clinical outcomes with left unilateral and sequential bilateral transcranial magnetic stimulation (TMS) treatment of major depressive disorder in a large patient registry. Brain Stimul 15(2):326–336, 2022 35074549

American Psychiatric Association: Practice guideline for the treatment of patients with major depressive disorder (revision). Am J Psychiatry 157(4 Suppl):1–45, 2000 10767867

American Psychiatric Association: Diagnostic and Statistical Manual of Mental Disorders, 5th Edition, Text Revision. Washington, DC, American Psychiatric Association, 2022

Avery DH, Isenberg KE, Sampson SM, et al: Transcranial magnetic stimulation in the acute treatment of major depressive disorder: clinical response in an open-label extension trial. J Clin Psychiatry 69(3):441–451, 2008 18294022

Beam W, Borckardt JJ, Reeves ST, et al: An efficient and accurate new method for locating the F3 position for prefrontal TMS applications. Brain Stimul 2(1):50–54, 2009 20539835

Benadhira R, Fanny T, Noomane B, et al: A randomized, sham-controlled study of maintenance rTMS for treatment-resistant depression (TRD). Psychiatry Res 258:226–233, 2017

Bersani FS, Minichino A, Enticott PG, et al: Deep transcranial magnetic stimulation as a treatment for psychiatric disorders: a comprehensive review. Eur Psychiatry 28(1):30–39, 2013 22559998

Bertocci MA, Afriyie-Agyemang Y, Rozovsky R, et al: Altered patterns of central executive, default mode and salience network activity and connectivity are associated with current and future depression risk in two independent young adult samples. Mol Psychiatry 28(3):1046–1056, 2023 36481935

Blumberger DM, Vila-Rodriguez F, Thorpe KE, et al: Effectiveness of theta burst versus high frequency repetitive transcranial magnetic stimulation in patients with depression (THREE-D): a randomized non-inferiority trial. Lancet 391(10131):1683–1692, 2018 29726344

Blumberger DM, Mulsant BH, Thorpe KE, et al: Effectiveness of standard sequential bilateral repetitive transcranial magnetic stimulation vs bilateral theta burst stimulation in older adults with depression: the FOUR-D randomized noninferiority clinical trial. JAMA Psychiatry 79(11):1065–1073, 2022 36129719

Brunoni AR, Chaimani A, Moffa AH, et al: Repetitive transcranial magnetic stimulation for the acute treatment of major depressive episodes: a systematic review with network meta-analysis. JAMA Psychiatry 74(2):143–152, 2017 28030740

Cardenas VA, Bhat JV, Horwege AM, et al: Anatomical and fMRI-network comparison of multiple DLPFC targeting strategies for repetitive transcranial magnetic stimulation treatment of depression. Brain Stimul 15(1):63–72, 2022 34767967

Carpenter LL, Janicak PG, Aaronson ST, et al: Transcranial magnetic stimulation (TMS) for major depression: a multisite, naturalistic, observational study of acute treatment outcomes in clinical practice. Depress Anxiety 29(7):587–596, 2012 22689344

Carpenter L, Aaronson S, Hutton TM, et al: Comparison of clinical outcomes with two transcranial magnetic stimulation treatment protocols for major depressive disorder. Brain Stimul 14(1):173–180, 2021 33346068

Cash RFH, Zalesky A, Thomson RH, et al: Subgenual functional connectivity predicts antidepressant treatment response to transcranial magnetic stimulation: independent validation and evaluation of personalization. Biol Psychiatry 86(2):e5–e7, 2019 30670304

Chatterjee B, Kumar N, Jha S: Role of repetitive transcranial magnetic stimulation in maintenance treatment of resistant depression. Indian J Psychol Med 34(3):286–289, 2012 23440309

Chen JJ, Liu Z, Zhu D, et al: Bilateral vs. unilateral repetitive transcranial magnetic stimulation in treating major depression: a meta-analysis of randomized controlled trials. Psychiatry Res 219(1):51–57, 2014 24889845

Cohen RB, Boggio PS, Fregni F: Risk factors for relapse after remission with repetitive transcranial magnetic stimulation for the treatment of depression. Depress Anxiety 26(7):682–688, 2009 19170101

Cole EJ, Stimpson KH, Bentzley BS, et al: Stanford accelerated intelligent neuromodulation therapy for treatment-resistant depression. Am J Psychiatry 177(8):716–726, 2020 32252538

Cole EJ, Phillips AL, Bentzley BS, et al: Stanford neuromodulation therapy (SNT): a double-blind randomized controlled trial. Am J Psychiatry 179(2):132–141, 2022 34711062

Connolly KR, Helmer A, Cristancho MA, et al: Effectiveness of transcranial magnetic stimulation in clinical practice post-FDA approval in the United States: results observed with the first 100 consecutive cases of depression at an academic medical center. J Clin Psychiatry 73(4):e567–e573, 2012 22579164

Cuijpers P, van Straten A, Warmerdam L, et al: Psychotherapy versus the combination of psychotherapy and pharmacotherapy in the treatment of depression: a meta-analysis. Depress Anxiety 26(3):279–288, 2009 19031487

Demirtas-Tatlidede A, Mechanic-Hamilton D, Press DZ, et al: An open-label, prospective study of repetitive transcranial magnetic stimulation (rTMS) in the long-term treatment of refractory depression: reproducibility and duration of the antidepressant effect in medication-free patients. J Clin Psychiatry 69(6):930–934, 2008 18505308

Deng ZD, Lisanby SH, Peterchev AV: Electric field depth-focality tradeoff in transcranial magnetic stimulation: simulation comparison of 50 coil designs. Brain Stimul 6(1):1–13, 2013 22483681

Di Lazzaro V, Dileone M, Pilato F, et al: Modulation of motor cortex neuronal networks by rTMS: comparison of local and remote effects of six different protocols of stimulation. J Neurophysiol 105(5):2150–2156, 2011 21346213

Dobson KS, Hollon SD, Dimidjian S, et al: Randomized trial of behavioral activation, cognitive therapy, and antidepressant medication in the prevention of relapse and recurrence in major depression. J Consult Clin Psychol 76(3):468–477, 2008 18540740

Dunner DL, Rush AJ, Russell JM, et al: Prospective, long-term, multicenter study of the naturalistic outcomes of patients with treatment-resistant depression. J Clin Psychiatry 67(5):688–695, 2006 16841617

Dunner DL, Aaronson ST, Sackeim HA, et al: A multisite, naturalistic, observational study of transcranial magnetic stimulation for patients with pharmacoresistant major depressive disorder: durability of benefit over a 1-year follow-up period. J Clin Psychiatry 75(12):1394–1401, 2014 25271871

Evans AC, Collins DL, Mills SR, et al: 3D statistical neuroanatomical models from 305 MRI volumes, in 1993 IEEE Conference Record Nuclear Science Symposium and Medical Imaging Conference. New York, IEEE, 1993, pp 1813–1817

Fava M, Davidson KG: Definition and epidemiology of treatment-resistant depression. Psychiatr Clin North Am 19(2):179–200, 1996 8827185

Filipčić I, Šimunović Filipčić I, Milovac Ž, et al: Efficacy of repetitive transcranial magnetic stimulation using a figure-8-coil or an H1-coil in treatment of major depressive disorder; a randomized clinical trial. J Psychiatr Res 114:113–119, 2019 31059991

First MB, Willams JBW, Karg RS, et al: Structured Clinical Interview for DSM-5 Disorders—Clinician Version (SCID-5-CV). Arlington, VA, American Psychiatric Association, 2016

Fitzgerald PB, Benitez J, de Castella A, et al: A randomized, controlled trial of sequential bilateral repetitive transcranial magnetic stimulation for treatment-resistant depression. Am J Psychiatry 163(1):88–94, 2006 16390894

Fitzgerald PB, Hoy K, McQueen S, et al: A randomized trial of rTMS targeted with MRI based neuro-navigation in treatment-resistant depression. Neuropsychopharmacology 34(5):1255–1262, 2009 19145228

Fitzgerald PB, Grace N, Hoy KE, et al: An open label trial of clustered maintenance rTMS for patients with refractory depression. Brain Stimul 6(3):292–297, 2013 22683273

Fitzgerald PB, Hoy KE, Reynolds J, et al: A pragmatic randomized controlled trial exploring the relationship between pulse number and response to repetitive transcranial magnetic stimulation treatment in depression. Brain Stimul 13(1):145–152, 2020 31521543

Fox MD, Buckner RL, White MP, et al: Efficacy of transcranial magnetic stimulation targets for depression is related to intrinsic functional connectivity with the subgenual cingulate. Biol Psychiatry 72(7):595–603, 2012 22658708

Fox MD, Liu H, Pascual-Leone A: Identification of reproducible individualized targets for treatment of depression with TMS based on intrinsic connectivity. Neuroimage 66:151–160, 2013 23142067

Galletly C, Gill S, Clarke P, et al: A randomized trial comparing repetitive transcranial magnetic stimulation given 3 days/week and 5 days/week for the treatment of major depression: is efficacy related to the duration of treatment or the number of treatments? Psychol Med 42(5):981–988, 2012 21910937

Gaynes BN, Warden D, Trivedi MH, et al: What did STAR*D teach us? Results from a large-scale, practical, clinical trial for patients with depression. Psychiatr Serv 60(11):1439–1445, 2009 19880458

Gaynes BN, Lloyd SW, Lux L, et al: Repetitive transcranial magnetic stimulation for treatment-resistant depression: a systematic review and meta-analysis. J Clin Psychiatry 75(5):477–489, quiz 489, 2014 24922485

Gellersen HM, Kedzior KK: Antidepressant outcomes of high-frequency repetitive transcranial magnetic stimulation (rTMS) with F8-coil and deep transcranial magnetic stimulation (DTMS) with H1-coil in major depression: a systematic review and meta-analysis. BMC Psychiatry 19(1):139, 2019 31064328

George MS, Lisanby SH, Avery D, et al: Daily left prefrontal transcranial magnetic stimulation therapy for major depressive disorder: a sham-controlled randomized trial. Arch Gen Psychiatry 67(5):507–516, 2010 20439832

George MS, Raman R, Benedek DM, et al: A two-site pilot randomized 3 day trial of high dose left prefrontal repetitive transcranial magnetic stimulation (rTMS) for suicidal inpatients. Brain Stimul 7(3):421–431, 2014 24731434

Greden JF: The burden of disease for treatment-resistant depression. J Clin Psychiatry 62(Suppl 16):26–31, 2001 11480881

Greenberg PE, Fournier AA, Sisitsky T, et al: The economic burden of adults with major depressive disorder in the United States (2010 and 2018). PharmacoEconomics 39(6):653–665, 2021 33950419

Grimm S, Beck J, Schuepbach D, et al: Imbalance between left and right dorsolateral prefrontal cortex in major depression is linked to negative emotional judgment: an fMRI study in severe major depressive disorder. Biol Psychiatry 63(4):369–376, 2008 17888408

Harel EV, Rabany L, Deutsch L, et al: H-coil repetitive transcranial magnetic stimulation for treatment resistant major depressive disorder: an 18-week continuation safety and feasibility study. World J Biol Psychiatry 15(4):298–306, 2014 22313023

Hasin DS, Sarvet AL, Meyers JL, et al: Epidemiology of adult DSM-5 major depressive disorder and its specifiers in the United States. JAMA Psychiatry 75(4):336–346, 2018 29450462

Holtzheimer PE III, McDonald WM, Mufti M, et al: Accelerated repetitive transcranial magnetic stimulation for treatment-resistant depression. Depress Anxiety 27(10):960–963, 2010 20734360

Hutton TM, Aaronson ST, Carpenter LL, et al: The anxiolytic and antidepressant effects of transcranial magnetic stimulation in patients with anxious depression. J Clin Psychiatry 84(1):22m14571, 2023 36630648

Iseger TA, Padberg F, Kenemans JL, et al: Neuro-cardiac-guided TMS (NCG-TMS): probing DLPFC-sgACC-vagus nerve connectivity using heart rate—first results. Brain Stimul 10(5):1006–1008, 2017 28545770

Iseger TA, Padberg F, Kenemans JL, et al: Neuro-cardiac-guided TMS (NCG TMS): a replication and extension study. Biol Psychol 162:108097, 2021 33895224

Iyer MB, Schleper N, Wassermann EM: Priming stimulation enhances the depressant effect of low-frequency repetitive transcranial magnetic stimulation. J Neurosci 23(34):10867–10872, 2003 14645480

Janicak PG, O'Reardon JP, Sampson SM, et al: Transcranial magnetic stimulation in the treatment of major depressive disorder: a comprehensive summary of safety experience from acute exposure, extended exposure, and during reintroduction treatment. J Clin Psychiatry 69(2):222–232, 2008 18232722

Janicak PG, Nahas Z, Lisanby SH, et al: Durability of clinical benefit with transcranial magnetic stimulation (TMS) in the treatment of pharmacoresistant major depression: assessment of relapse during a 6-month, multisite, open-label study. Brain Stimul 3(4):187–199, 2010 20965447

Janicak PG, Dunner DL, Aaronson ST, et al: Transcranial magnetic stimulation (TMS) for major depression: a multisite, naturalistic, observational study of quality of life outcome measures in clinical practice. CNS Spectr 18(6):322–332, 2013 23895940

Kalin NH: Spanning treatment modalities: psychotherapy, psychopharmacology, and neuromodulation. Am J Psychiatry 179(2):75–78, 2022 35105160

Kaur M, Michael JA, Hoy KE, et al: Investigating high- and low-frequency neurocardiac-guided TMS for probing the frontal vagal pathway. Brain Stimul 13(3):931–938, 2020 32205066

Keller MB, Trivedi MH, Thase ME, et al: The Prevention of Recurrent Episodes of Depression with Venlafaxine for Two Years (PREVENT) study: outcomes from the 2-year and combined maintenance phases. J Clin Psychiatry 68(8):1246–1256, 2007 17854250

Levkovitz Y, Isserles M, Padberg F, et al: Efficacy and safety of deep transcranial magnetic stimulation for major depression: a prospective multicenter randomized controlled trial. World Psychiatry 14(1):64–73, 2015 25655160

Li CT, Cheng CM, Chen MH, et al: Antidepressant efficacy of prolonged intermittent theta burst stimulation monotherapy for recurrent depression and comparison of methods for coil positioning: a randomized, double-blind, sham-controlled study. Biol Psychiatry 87(5):443–450, 2020 31563272

Lim GY, Tam WW, Lu Y, et al: Prevalence of depression in the community from 30 countries between 1994 and 2014. Sci Rep 8(1):1–10, 2018 29434331

Mayberg HS: Modulating dysfunctional limbic-cortical circuits in depression: towards development of brain-based algorithms for diagnosis and optimised treatment. Br Med Bull 65(1):193–207, 2003 12697626

McAllister-Williams RH, Arango C, Blier P, et al: The identification, assessment and management of difficult-to-treat depression: an international consensus statement. J Affect Disord 267:264–282, 2020 32217227

Mehta S, Konstantinou G, Weissman CR, et al: The effect of repetitive transcranial magnetic stimulation on suicidal ideation in treatment-resistant depression: a meta-analysis. J Clin Psychiatry 83(2):21r13969, 2022 35044731

Mir-Moghtadaei A, Caballero R, Fried P, et al: Concordance between BeamF3 and MRI-neuronavigated target sites for repetitive transcranial magnetic stimulation of the left dorsolateral prefrontal cortex. Brain Stimul 8(5):965–973, 2015 26115776

Nordentoft M, Mortensen PB, Pedersen CB: Absolute risk of suicide after first hospital contact in mental disorder. Arch Gen Psychiatry 68(10):1058–1064, 2019

O'Reardon JP, Blumner KH, Peshek AD, et al: Long-term maintenance therapy for major depressive disorder with rTMS. J Clin Psychiatry 66(12):1524–1528, 2005 16401152

O'Reardon JP, Solvason HB, Janicak PG, et al: Efficacy and safety of transcranial magnetic stimulation in the acute treatment of major depression: a multisite randomized controlled trial. Biol Psychiatry 62(11):1208–1216, 2007 17573044

Pallanti S, Bernardi S, Di Rollo A, et al: Unilateral low frequency versus sequential bilateral repetitive transcranial magnetic stimulation: is simpler better for treatment of resistant depression? Neuroscience 167(2):323–328, 2010 20144692

Pell GS, Harmelech T, Zibman S, et al: Efficacy of deep TMS with the H1 coil for anxious depression. J Clin Med 11(4):1015, 2022 35207288

Perera T, George MS, Grammer G, et al: The Clinical TMS Society consensus review and treatment recommendations for TMS therapy for major depressive disorder. Brain Stimul 9(3):336–346, 2016 27090022

Philip NS, Dunner DL, Dowd SM, et al: Can medication free, treatment-resistant, depressed patients who initially respond to TMS be maintained off medications? A prospective, 12-month multisite randomized pilot study. Brain Stimul 9(2):251–257, 2016 26708778

Pigott HE, Kim T, Xu C, et al: What are the treatment remission, response and extent of improvement rates after up to four trials of antidepressant therapies in real-world depressed patients? A reanalysis of the STAR*D study's patient-level data with fidelity to the original research protocol. BMJ Open 13(7):e063095, 2023 37491091

Prudic J, Olfson M, Marcus SC, et al: Effectiveness of electroconvulsive therapy in community settings. Biol Psychiatry 55(3):301–312, 2004 14744473

Richieri R, Guedj E, Michel P, et al: Maintenance transcranial magnetic stimulation reduces depression relapse: a propensity-adjusted analysis. J Affect Disord 151(1):129–135, 2013 23790811

Rush AJ, Trivedi MH, Wisniewski SR, et al: Acute and longer-term outcomes in depressed outpatients requiring one or several treatment steps: a STAR*D report. Am J Psychiatry 163(11):1905–1917, 2020

Sackeim HA: Acute continuation and maintenance treatment of major depressive episodes with transcranial magnetic stimulation. Brain Stimul 9(3):313–319, 2016 27052475

Sackeim HA, Aaronson ST, Carpenter LL, et al: Clinical outcomes in a large registry of patients with major depressive disorder treated with transcranial magnetic stimulation. J Affect Disord 277:65–74, 2020 32799106

Schutter DJ: Antidepressant efficacy of high-frequency transcranial magnetic stimulation over the left dorsolateral prefrontal cortex in double-blind sham-controlled designs: a meta-analysis. Psychol Med 39(1):65–75, 2009 18447962

Schutter DJ: Quantitative review of the efficacy of slow-frequency magnetic brain stimulation in major depressive disorder. Psychol Med 40(11):1789–1795, 2010 20102670

Senova S, Cotovio G, Pascual-Leone A, et al: Durability of antidepressant response to repetitive transcranial magnetic stimulation: systematic review and meta-analysis. Brain Stimul 12(1):119–128, 2019 30344109

Serafini G, Pompili M, Belvederi Murri M, et al: The effects of repetitive transcranial magnetic stimulation on cognitive performance in treatment-resistant depression: a systematic review. Neuropsychobiology 71(3):125–139, 2015 25925699

Sheehan DV, Lecrubier Y, Sheehan KH, et al: The Mini-International Neuropsychiatric Interview (M.I.N.I.): the development and validation of a structured diagnostic psychiatric interview for DSM-IV and ICD-10. J Clin Psychiatry 59(Suppl 20):22–33, quiz 34–57, 1998 9881538

Siddiqi SH, Trapp NT, Hacker CD, et al: Repetitive transcranial magnetic stimulation with resting-state network targeting for treatment-resistant depression in traumatic brain injury: a randomized, controlled, double-blinded pilot study. J Neurotrauma 36(8):1361–1374, 2019 30381997

Siddiqi SH, Taylor SF, Cooke D, et al: Distinct symptom-specific treatment targets for circuit-based neuromodulation. Am J Psychiatry 177(5):435–446, 2020 32160765

Slotema CW, Blom JD, Hoek HW, et al: Should we expand the toolbox of psychiatric treatment methods to include repetitive transcranial magnetic stimulation (rTMS)? A meta-analysis of the efficacy of rTMS in psychiatric disorders. J Clin Psychiatry 71(7):873–884, 2010 20361902

Sonmez AI, Camsari DD, Nandakumar AL, et al: Accelerated TMS for depression: a systematic review and meta-analysis. Psychiatry Res 273:770–781, 2019 31207865

Spielmans GI, Berman MI, Linardatos E, et al: Adjunctive atypical antipsychotic treatment for major depressive disorder: a meta-analysis of depression, quality of life, and safety outcomes. PLoS Med 10(3):e1001403, 2013

Tendler A, Goerigk S, Zibman S, et al: Deep TMS H1 coil treatment for depression: results from a large post marketing data analysis. Psychiatry Res 324:115179, 2023 37030054

Trapp N, Pace B, Neisewander B, et al: A randomized trial comparing Beam F3 and 5.5 cm targeting in rTMS treatment of depression demonstrates similar effectiveness. Brain Stimul 16(5):1392–1400, 2023 37714408

Voigt JD, Leuchter AF, Carpenter LL: Theta burst stimulation for the acute treatment of major depressive disorder: a systematic review and meta-analysis. Transl Psychiatry 11(1):330, 2021 34050123

Wang WL, Wang SY, Hung HY, et al: Safety of transcranial magnetic stimulation in unipolar depression: a systematic review and meta-analysis of randomized-controlled trials. J Affect Disord 301:400–425, 2022 35032510

Warden D, Rush AJ, Trivedi MH, et al: The STAR*D project results: a comprehensive review of findings. Curr Psychiatry Rep 9(6):449–459, 2007 18221624

Weissman CR, Blumberger DM, Brown PE, et al: Bilateral repetitive transcranial magnetic stimulation decreases suicidal ideation in depression. J Clin Psychiatry 79(3):17m11692, 2018 29701939

Williams NR, Sudheimer KD, Bentzley BS, et al: High-dose spaced theta-burst TMS as a rapid-acting antidepressant in highly refractory depression. Brain 141(3):e18, 2018 29415152

Wilson S, Croarkin PE, Aaronson ST, et al: Systematic review of preservation TMS that includes continuation, maintenance, relapse-prevention, and rescue TMS. J Affect Disord 296:79–88, 2022 34592659

World Health Organization: The ICD-10 Classification of Mental and Behavioural Disorders: Clinical Descriptions and Diagnostic Guidelines, Vol 1. Geneva, World Health Organization, 1992

World Health Organization: Depressive disorder (depression). March 31, 2023. Available at: https://www.who.int/news-room/fact-sheets/detail/depression. Accessed September 22, 2024.

Zhdanava M, Pilon D, Ghelerter I, et al: The economic burden of treatment-resistant depression in the United States: a retrospective database analysis. J Manag Care Spec Pharm 27(4):516–527, 2021

Integrating Pharmacotherapy and Psychotherapy With Transcranial Magnetic Stimulation for Major Depressive Disorder

Mehmet E. Dokucu, M.D., Ph.D.
Richard A. Bermudes, M.D.
Philip G. Janicak, M.D.

In managing any illness, a clinician should initially consider a monotherapy that yields high efficacy with comparatively few adverse effects (AEs). Complex psychiatric disorders, however, often require a multimodal treatment approach to improve outcomes, especially for patients with treatment-resistant depression (TRD). In this chapter, we review integrat-

63

ing pharmacological and nonpharmacological interventions with transcranial magnetic stimulation (TMS), focusing on TRD. Several reports support a combined approach, ranging from case reports to randomized controlled trials (RCTs). Thus, rather than replacing partially effective medications and psychological treatments in clinical practice, TMS is combined with them to enhance outcomes. We first review the knowledge base and recommended clinical practices for using TMS in combination with pharmacotherapy for acute treatment, sequentially when transitioning from acute TMS therapy to maintenance medication therapy, and again in combination if TMS reintroduction is needed during the maintenance period. Then we review various types of psychotherapy and how these therapies can be integrated with TMS.

Combining TMS With Medication

The high prevalence of TRD was an essential impetus in TMS development. To adequately demonstrate the efficacy of TMS in treating TRD, the pivotal trials included patients who received monotherapy TMS or sham TMS. On the basis of those results, the FDA cleared TMS for treating major depressive disorder (MDD) in patients who had experienced one or more failed antidepressant medication trials. In clinical practice, however, most patients continue taking psychotropic medications while receiving an acute course of TMS. Also, after completion of the acute course, the most common maintenance strategy uses antidepressant medication(s) with or without reintroduction of TMS for an impending relapse. In support of this practice, the consensus review of the Clinical TMS Society states that "TMS therapy can be administered with or without the concomitant administration of antidepressant or other psychotropic medications. There is no evidence of an increased risk of adverse events by combining medications with TMS" (Perera et al. 2016, p. 344). According to a survey of Clinical TMS Society members, most practitioners recommend continuing medications during acute TMS therapy and refraining from medication changes during the acute course (Perera et al. 2016).

The choice of medication to combine with TMS for optimal outcomes remains problematic. Our understanding of the mechanism of action of device-based treatments such as electroconvulsive therapy, deep brain stimulation, and TMS is still evolving (see Chapter 1, "Basic Principles of Transcranial Magnetic Stimulation"). Thus, because of the heterogeneity of depressive syndromes and the lack of consistent biological markers, no treatments are based on well-described disease mechanisms. This lack of understanding of the mechanism of action is true for other forms of therapy as well; as a result, it is impossible to make precise statements about the interaction between TMS and pharmacotherapy when administered concurrently or sequentially during the treatment of MDD. Because the uniqueness of TMS may lie in its ability to target specific neural networks, we hope to develop potential neurocircuit-based therapeutic and diagnostic approaches to disorders such as MDD (e.g., Siddiqi et al. 2022; see Chapter 2, "Transcranial Magnetic Stimulation Therapy for Major Depression"). Thus, as described in the "Augmentation Studies Combining Medication and TMS" section, combining medications and/or psychotherapy with TMS may improve benefits as a result of augmentation through additive or synergistic mechanisms of action.

Augmentation Studies Combining Medication and TMS

Acute Studies

Many early TMS studies were augmentation trials. For example, Conca et al. (1996) administered 10 sessions of low-frequency TMS to 12 patients taking antidepressants and compared their results with those of 12 patients who received only medication. Statistically significant changes in scores on the Hamilton Depression Rating Scale (HDRS) favored TMS augmentation after three sessions ($P<0.003$), with improvement being even greater after the tenth session ($P<0.001$). The same research group performed a brief course of 10-day add-on TMS in 12 inpatients and reported that 8 subjects (66.7%) responded to the treatment as assessed by HDRS change scores (Conca et al. 2000). They also observed an earlier onset of response in the TMS group (statistical analysis not made available) and proposed that a shorter duration of the index depressive episode may be a positive predictor of treatment response. In an open-label study, Berlim et al. (2014) used deep TMS to augment medications. Seventeen outpatients with severe TRD received 4 weeks of daily high-frequency deep TMS. On the basis of HDRS change scores, the remission rate was 41.2% at week 5, and the response rate was 70.6%. Furthermore, suicidality ($P<0.019$), anxiety ($P<0.001$), and quality-of-life ($P<0.03$) scores also were significantly improved from baseline.

Carpenter et al. (2012) reported the results of a large open-label, naturalistic, acute trial in 42 practice settings to inform clinicians using TMS. The primary outcome measure was the Clinical Global Impression—Severity of Illness Scale (CGI-S) change score. Secondary outcomes were change scores on the Inventory of Depressive Symptomatology—Self-

Report (IDS-SR) and the 9-item Patient Health Questionnaire (PHQ-9). Nearly all patients continued taking their current psychiatric medications. On the basis of the CGI-S change scores at the end of acute TMS therapy, more than half of the patients met response criteria, and approximately one-third achieved remission. Notably, AEs did not increase with combined TMS and psychotropics.

In an RCT, Su et al. (2005) studied 30 Chinese patients with TRD in which a 10-session TMS course was added to ongoing medications. Ten participants were assigned to one of three groups, receiving 20-Hz TMS, 5-Hz TMS, or sham TMS. On the basis of HDRS change scores, response rates for patients in the two active TMS arms were superior to those for patients receiving the sham procedure ($P<0.01$).

An 8-week multicenter, U.S.-based, randomized open-label study entitled Augmentation Versus Switch: Comparative Effectiveness Research Trial for Antidepressant Incomplete and Non-responders With Treatment Resistant Depression (ASCERTAIN-TRD) evaluated patients with TRD undergoing TMS versus taking aripiprazole as an augmentation to ongoing, stable, and adequate antidepressant therapy (Papakostas et al. 2024). The trial comprised three open-label active treatment arms consisting of aripiprazole augmentation (5 mg/day starting dosage; 15 mg/day maximum), standard 10-Hz TMS augmentation, and a switch to a serotonin-norepinephrine reuptake inhibitor (SNRI) (i.e., venlafaxine extended-release or duloxetine). The primary outcome was the Montgomery-Åsberg Depression Rating Scale (MADRS) change score; a secondary outcome was the self-rated Symptoms of Depression Questionnaire (SDQ) change score. Two hundred and thirty-five participants completed the study. Multiple comparisons were made between treatments, with the TMS augmentation arm ($n=61$) outperforming the aripiprazole augmentation ($n=83$) and SNRI switch ($n=91$) arms in all comparisons (i.e., MADRS and SDQ change scores, MADRS response, and remission rates). Statistical significance was achieved for the MADRS change score, with TMS augmentation being superior to the SNRI switch (−17.3 vs. −13.1), indicating a medium to large effect size approximately equal to Cohen's d of 0.51 ($P<0.01$). In addition, SDQ change scores with aripiprazole augmentation were superior to those for the SNRI switch (37.5 vs. 32.8), indicating a small effect size approximately equal to Cohen's d of 0.21 ($P<0.002$). Although TMS augmentation yielded a larger decrease in the SDQ change score (−42.4 vs. 32.8), it was not statistically significant ($P<0.05$) at the prespecified significance level of $P<0.03$.

Although TMS is not FDA cleared for treating bipolar disorder, many patients receive it off-label for the depressed phase of their disorder (see

Chapter 4, "Transcranial Magnetic Stimulation for the Treatment of Other Mood Disorders"). A small add-on safety and feasibility trial with TMS in patients ($N=19$) with bipolar depression taking psychotropic medication found a significant decrease from baseline HDRS scores ($P<0.001$). Treatment was well tolerated regarding headache and overall discomfort, and no significant changes were seen in cognitive functioning or mood switches. One patient had a short generalized seizure without complications (Harel et al. 2011).

Meta-analyses of TMS Acute Augmentation Studies

Liu et al. (2014) conducted a meta-analysis of sham-controlled clinical trials to clarify whether TMS enhances the efficacy of antidepressants in patients with TRD. Seven randomized trials met the investigators' inclusion criteria, with a total sample size of 279 (171 active TMS patients and 108 sham TMS patients). Response rates and number needed to treat were chosen as the primary outcomes, and remission rates, change from baseline HDRS scores, and dropout rate were used as secondary outcomes. The pooled response and remission rates for the TMS and sham groups were 46.6% and 22.1%, respectively; the pooled OR was 5.12 (95% CI=2.11–12.45; $z=3.60$; $P<0.03$), and the associated number needed to treat was 3.4. The TMS group achieved a significant reduction in HDRS score compared with the sham group; the pooled standardized mean difference of change from baseline was 0.86 (95% CI=0.57–1.15; $z=5.75$; $P<0.001$). Only two RCTs reported the number of remitters at the end of blinded TMS treatment; both found a significant difference between the active and the sham groups in achieving remission. The results of an earlier meta-analysis (six studies, $N=392$) were comparable (Berlim et al. 2013). Furthermore, the authors commented that high-frequency TMS may accelerate the time to antidepressant response.

Maintenance Augmentation Studies

The pivotal monotherapy TMS trial that led to FDA clearance of the first device to treat MDD included a 6-month durability-of-effect phase. During this period, TMS could be reintroduced as an augmentation to maintenance antidepressant monotherapy. Of the patients with predefined worsening of depression for 2 consecutive weeks, 84% (32 of 38) benefited from the reintroduction of TMS (requiring an average of ~14 sessions), with no increase in AEs (Janicak et al. 2010; O'Reardon et al. 2007).

Phase III of the randomized sham-controlled National Institute of Mental Health–sponsored Optimization of TMS for Depression (OPT-

TMS) study involved medicated and unmedicated patients who achieved remission after Phases I and II. Although participants were followed up for 6 months, only the 3-month analysis was performed because of attrition. Approximately half of the patients who achieved remission took medication, typically venlafaxine or nortriptyline combined with lithium or lamotrigine. Medicated and unmedicated patient groups showed no significant difference in clinical outcome at the 3-month follow-up. Fifty-eight percent of the participants were still in remission at 3 months, and 13.5% of the patients had relapsed. The average time to relapse was 7.2 weeks (Mantovani et al. 2012).

The largest maintenance study extended to 12 months and included 275 patients with TRD at the end of the acute phase (as summarized in the "Acute Studies" subsection) (Carpenter et al. 2012; Dunner et al. 2014). At the end of the study, 120 patients achieved response or remission and were offered maintenance medication or naturalistic follow-up with the choice of reintroduction TMS therapy if symptoms worsened. Throughout the 52-week follow-up, 62% of the participants maintained at least a response status. Dunner and colleagues concluded that TMS could achieve durability of benefit in a statistically significant ($P < 0.0001$) and clinically meaningful way. Of note, 32.5% of the participants required a mean number of 16.2 sessions of reintroduction TMS within 1 month of initiating their maintenance phase. As in the acute-phase naturalistic study, almost all patients took concomitant medications, with the median number being one medication for remitters and two for the rest of the cohort. No meaningful associations were reported between medication use and categorical outcomes.

Clinical Considerations When Combining TMS With Medications

Assessment of Medication Timeline, Benefits, and Adverse Effects

During the initial TMS consultation, the clinician should obtain a comprehensive history of antidepressant medications. Although cumbersome, the Antidepressant Treatment History Form is one tool that can help clinicians gather this information (Sackeim 2001). Although this history is taken primarily to establish the level of treatment resistance, the data can also help inform pharmacotherapy treatment decisions while TMS therapy is in progress. All concomitant psychotropic medications should be carefully categorized as partially helpful or not helpful. Medications that are not at least partially helpful should be sequentially tapered and stopped. Medications contributing to AEs (e.g., weight gain) that are not helpful should be tapered first. Ideally, a patient's medication regimen should be stable for at least 2–4 weeks before they start TMS; this preparation allows the physician to assess the AEs and response to TMS specifically.

Obtaining a list of all current medications, their dosages, and the duration of treatment is critical to understanding and minimizing the risk of seizures. In addition, some medications (e.g., benzodiazepines and high-dose anticonvulsants) may diminish TMS's efficacy by increasing neuronal circuit activation thresholds (Li et al. 2004). Finally, if patients report AEs that do not commonly occur during TMS, full knowledge of current medications and their timeline may help clinicians identify the source more accurately.

Risk for Symptom Worsening With Medication Changes and Complex Polypharmacy During TMS

Some patients would like to discontinue their current psychiatric medications when they present for a consultation session and will seek the opinion of the TMS clinician. Medication-related AEs and a lack of confidence in the effectiveness are the most common reasons for discontinuation. The TMS clinician can formulate an opinion only with a detailed understanding of current medications and the temporal relationship with symptom changes. Furthermore, if the TMS clinician is not the patient's primary mental health care provider, direct communication with that provider is essential in formulating a plan about any medication changes that may enhance TMS's efficacy, decrease the risk for AEs, or both. Reviewing records and communicating with the patient's primary treatment team and family help clarify specific medications' effectiveness. Patients may not see their primary psychiatric providers during the TMS course, which increases the importance of the TMS clinician being familiar with the medication regimen and response history.

Often, patients with difficult-to-treat depression are taking multiple medications that accumulate over time because of concerns about symptoms worsening with tapering. In this context, clinicians can take advantage of the efficacy of TMS as a monotherapy to remove suspect medications, thus simplifying complex polypharmacy regimens and enhancing safety and tolerability (Mojtabai and Olfson 2020).

Medications That May Increase TMS-Related Seizures

Table 3–1 lists the Safety of TMS Consensus Group guidelines for medications that may worsen the seizure risk associated with TMS treatment

(Rossi et al. 2009, 2021). Although many antidepressants can lower the seizure threshold, bupropion carries a more prominent warning regarding this potential. Hence, we review it in more detail.

Bupropion, compared with other medications, has lower risks of sexual dysfunction and weight gain and therefore is commonly prescribed as a monotherapy or augmenting agent for depressed patients. However, it carries an increased seizure risk in special populations (i.e., those with eating disorders or seizure history) and may alter the motor threshold (Mufti et al. 2010). Some TMS candidates and their referring clinicians may ask whether it is safe to continue bupropion during treatment. Regarding this issue, one systematic literature review (Dobek et al. 2015) identified 25 TMS-induced seizures between 1980 and 2015, none of which were related to taking bupropion. One patient whose TMS-induced seizure was reported to the FDA was concomitantly taking bupropion, sertraline, and amphetamine. Dobek and colleagues stated that the rare occurrence of seizures during TMS did not point to a specific antidepressant such as bupropion. In support, Janicak et al. (2008) reported on 34 patients taking bupropion who underwent more than 1,000 TMS treatments without a seizure event.

The updated safety recommendations for TMS downgrade warnings regarding contributions from psychiatric medications to seizures to negligible (Rossi et al. 2009, 2021) on the basis of more recent surveys (e.g., Lerner et al. 2019). Nevertheless, we include Table 3–1 from the previous edition as an information resource.

Clinical Vignette 1

A 27-year-old resident physician presented for TMS therapy to manage his 4-month treatment-resistant major depressive episode and comorbid migraines. A comprehensive medication history was obtained, and the patient's primary psychiatrist was contacted for verification. He was taking bupropion extended-release 450 mg/day, initiated after his poor tolerance of two selective serotonin reuptake inhibitors and one SNRI because of sexual dysfunction and increased appetite and associated weight gain. The bupropion daily dosage was titrated from 150 mg to 450 mg because of a gradual but slight improvement of his depressive symptoms. Even at this dosage, however, he continued to experience functional impairment and dosage-related worsening of his migraines. He then received left dorsolateral prefrontal cortex high-frequency (10-Hz) TMS therapy, and over the course of 2 weeks, his bupropion dosage was tapered to 150 mg, with complete resolution of his migraines. He continued TMS for another 4 weeks, ultimately achieving complete remission of depressive symptoms, with a final IDS-SR score of 6 (down from a baseline score of 53). Furthermore, the patient experienced no significant AEs with bupropion plus TMS.

Table 3–1. Concomitant medications and seizure risk safety classifications, adapted from Safety of TMS Consensus Group guidelines

Strong risk with intake of agent (perform TMS with particular caution)	Relative risk with intake of agent (perform TMS with caution)	Relative risk with withdrawal from agent (perform TMS with caution)
Antidepressants	Antidepressants and mood stabilizers	Anticonvulsants and mood stabilizers
Imipramine	Mianserin	Benzodiazepines
Amitriptyline	Fluoxetine	Lamotrigine
Doxepin	Fluvoxamine	Divalproex
Nortriptyline	Paroxetine	Phenytoin
Maprotiline	Sertraline	Sedatives and anxiolytics
Amphetamines	Citalopram	Benzodiazepines
Antipsychotics	Mirtazapine	Barbiturates
Chlorpromazine	Reboxetine	Meprobamate
Clozapine	Bupropion	Chloral hydrate
Drugs of abuse	Lithium	Drugs of abuse
Alcohol	Antipsychotics	Alcohol
Amphetamines	Fluphenazine	Benzodiazepines
Ketamine	Pimozide	Barbiturates
Phencyclidine	Haloperidol	
Cocaine	Olanzapine	
γ-Hydroxybutyrate	Quetiapine	
3,4-Methylenedioxymethamphetamine (MDMA, Ecstasy)	Aripiprazole	
	Ziprasidone	
	Risperidone	

Table 3-1. Concomitant medications and seizure risk safety classifications, adapted from Safety of TMS Consensus Group guidelines *(continued)*

Strong risk with intake of agent (perform TMS with particular caution)	Relative risk with intake of agent (perform TMS with caution)	Relative risk with withdrawal from agent (perform TMS with caution)
Other	Other	
Foscarnet	Chloroquine	
Theophylline	Mefloquine	
Ganciclovir	Imipenem	
	Penicillin	
	Ampicillin	
	Cephalosporins	
	Metronidazole	
	Isoniazid	
	Levofloxacin	
	Cyclosporine	
	Chlorambucil	
	Vincristine	
	Methotrexate	
	Cytosine arabinoside	
	Bis-chloroethylnitrosourea	
	Anticholinergics	
	Antihistamines	
	Sympathomimetics	

Note. TMS=transcranial magnetic stimulation.

Risk for Switching or Activation When Combining TMS With Antidepressant Medications

As with antidepressant monotherapy (Harada et al. 2008), TMS combined with antidepressant medication may carry a risk of activation (i.e., anxiety, agitation, insomnia, irritability, or restlessness) without induction of a full-blown hypomanic or manic episode (Harada et al. 2008). Philip et al. (2015) operationally defined symptoms as being present when patient-reported anxiety, insomnia, or psychomotor agitation emerged (or worsened relative to baseline levels) during TMS therapy. They reviewed records for patients ($n=98$) who received 15 or more acute TMS treatments while taking psychotropic medications; 28% developed clinically significant activation, necessitating a switch in the TMS stimulation protocol from 10 Hz to 5 Hz. For the most part, patients were similar in terms of demographic variables. However, patients who had more activation, requiring a switch to 5 Hz, were more likely to have comorbid anxiety compared with patients in the 10-Hz group (85% vs. 51%; $\chi^2=9.7$; $P<0.002$). We have not found systematic studies considering whether concomitant medications play a role in such AEs. Moreover, the potential switching effect of antidepressants in patients with unipolar depression is poorly understood.

Medications That May Compromise TMS Efficacy

The concern that the concomitant use of benzodiazepines may compromise efficacy and/or alter TMS dose requirements did not surface in the earlier literature (Ziemann 2013). However, several subsequent reports suggested that clinicians may want to lower or taper these medications before TMS therapy. For example, Hunter et al. (2019) reported in their retrospective observational study that among patients undergoing TMS therapy for depression, concomitant benzodiazepine use lowered response rates compared with those of nonusers ($n=72$; 16.4% vs. 35.5%; $P<0.008$) after 6 weeks of treatment. This finding did not depend on the severity of anxiety symptoms. A similar association was reported by Kaster et al. (2019) in a secondary analysis of an intermittent theta burst stimulation (iTBS) TMS noninferiority trial (Blumberger et al. 2018). Kaster et al. (2019) found that lack of benzodiazepine use was significantly associated with a more rapid response to iTBS ($n=73$; OR for rapid response$=0.40$; 95% CI$=0.18$–0.90; $P<0.005$). In another retrospective study, Deppe et al. (2021) reported that patients ($n=73$) taking lorazepam had an 18% response rate to TMS compared with a 38% response rate among nonusers (HDRS, $n=176$; $P<0.002$). Conversely, in a post hoc analysis of pooled data from two accelerated TMS clinical trials (left-sided high frequency and iTBS), no difference was found between benzodiazepine users ($n=64$) and nonusers ($n=121$) on the basis of the MADRS change scores (−27 vs. −27; $P<0.99$) or response rates (25% vs. 24.8%; $P<0.98$) (Fitzgerald et al. 2020). Of note, care must be taken not to abruptly stop benzodiazepines, which can increase seizure risk, particularly in patients with epilepsy.

Medications to Minimize Risks Associated With TMS

Severe insomnia, sometimes resulting in sleep deprivation, can significantly increase seizure risk during TMS therapy. This risk can be reduced by treating insomnia with ramelteon, trazodone, zolpidem, zaleplon, or eszopiclone. If available, cognitive-behavioral therapy (CBT) for insomnia may be the preferred option.

Some patients with significant anxiety and/or restlessness may find sitting still during a TMS session challenging. Such patients can be premedicated with low doses of quetiapine, diphenhydramine, or hydroxyzine if their restlessness is not responsive to changes in their scheduled medications.

It is acceptable but not common for patients to take over-the-counter nonsteroidal anti-inflammatory medications before their sessions to decrease scalp discomfort or headaches. More severe discomfort may occasionally require local anesthetics (e.g., topical skin preparations).

Enhancing TMS Outcomes With Medications

Using medications to augment the antidepressant efficacy of TMS is an exciting development. Examples include D-cycloserine, psychostimulants, and ketamine (Korchounov and Ziemann 2011). Synaptic plasticity and activation of the N-methyl-D-aspartate receptors in long-term potentiation appear to be integral to TMS's antidepressant effects (Brown et al. 2022). In this context, D-cycloserine, an N-methyl-D-aspartate receptor agonist, was studied as an augmentation agent to enhance the effects of TMS in patients with MDD (Cole et al. 2022). The investigators recruited 50 participants with major depression into a single-site, 4-week RCT with two arms: iTBS plus placebo and iTBS plus 100 mg of D-cycloserine (taken 60 minutes before treatment). The primary outcome was the MADRS change score, which decreased by 16.16 points in the D-cycloserine group ($n=25$) versus 10.20 points in the placebo group ($P<0.007$). Moreover, clinical response rates were higher in the iTBS plus D-cycloserine group than in the iTBS plus placebo group (73.9% vs. 29.3%), as were clinical remission rates (39.1% vs. 4.2%). No serious adverse events occurred.

Psychostimulants enhance monoaminergic signaling in neural pathways. A retrospective, observational study of medications taken by University of California, Los Angeles, clinic patients reported that by as early as week 2 and then at 6 weeks of TMS therapy, those who also received psychostimulants improved significantly more than the psychostimulant nonusers (Hunter et al. 2019). These effects were significant after controlling for baseline variables, including age, overall symptom severity, and severity of anxiety symptoms. Response rates at week 6 were higher in psychostimulant users than in nonusers (39.2% vs. 22.0%; $P<0.02$). In a subsequent analysis, Wilke et al. (2022) examined the psychostimulant data in greater detail, looking at effects on total IDS-SR (30 items) score, as well as subscales examining separate domains of "mood/cognition," "anxiety/arousal," and "sleep"; differences among psychostimulant medication categories; and dose-response relationships. On the basis of the IDS-SR, symptom severity was significantly lower in psychostimulant users than in nonusers over the course of treatment (−13.9 vs. −9.56; $P<0.03$), and response rates were greater than 39.2% versus 22.0%, respectively ($P<0.02$). In addition to overall improvement, the psychostimulant group had more improvement in mood cognition and sleep but not in anxiety/arousal. Lower doses (<20 mg) of lisdexamfetamine or dextroamphetamine produced better outcomes than higher doses.

Use of ketamine to augment TMS effects is another potential option. However, no systematic studies were identified. Two case reports suggested that adding ketamine may mitigate resistance to TMS (Elkrief et al. 2022) and is safe and beneficial (Best et al. 2019).

Rationale for Combining TMS and Psychotherapy

Evidence suggests that brain plasticity in response to stimulation depends on the state of the brain or the activation of the circuit during stimulation (Gersner et al. 2011; Vedeniapin et al. 2010). Thus, combined with different concurrent psychotherapies, TMS may synergistically improve clinical outcomes compared with a stand-alone treatment. Additionally, specific tasks or protocols could induce an *optimal brain state* before, during, or after stimulation, leading to improved outcomes (Bajbouj and Padberg 2014; Silvanto et al. 2008, 2018).

Preclinical animal and human studies support this notion. In an animal study, high-frequency stimulation caused a profound effect on neuroplasticity markers, which increased in awake animals and decreased in anesthetized animals (Gersner et al. 2011). Isserles et al. (2011) showed that the antidepressant outcome of TMS treatment is affected by a cognitive-emotional procedure performed during stimulation. Positive or negative cognitive-emotional reactivation was administered to patients while they received 4 weeks of acute TMS and 4 weeks of maintenance therapy. Depression scores did not significantly improve in the negatively reactivated group, signifying that negative cognitive-emotional reactivation may disrupt the therapeutic effects of TMS. These results suggest that psychotherapy during TMS treatment sessions may affect brain state and, ultimately, the response to treatment.

Psychotherapy and mindfulness meditation induce neuroplastic changes in brain function and structure (see Figure 3–1) (Chiesa et al. 2013; Sheline et al. 2017; Tang et al. 2015). Because both TMS and psychotherapy have this capacity, engaging the brain via psychotherapy during a TMS session may magnify the benefits and enhance the durability of both treatments. Furthermore, while undergoing TMS, a more engaged brain (i.e., during psychotherapy) may be more receptive to the benefits of TMS than a less active brain (i.e., while watching television). Thus, combining the two interventions may have a complementary or synergistic effect by modulating mood circuits.

Although TMS may prime and augment psychotherapy if these treatments are administered in succession (*offline* therapy), it is also practical to coadminister psychotherapy during TMS sessions (*online* therapy) because patients come to the clinic 5 days/week and, on average, are in a treatment session for 25–45 minutes. Figure 3–2 provides an overview of administering TMS with psychotherapy.

Clinical Vignette 2

A 57-year-old man was receiving sequential bilateral TMS for severe, recurrent TRD and comorbid generalized anxiety disorder. He previously underwent two courses of CBT and multiple antidepressant medication trials, each of which was partially effective. Throughout his TMS treatment (42 sessions total), he received concurrent psychotherapy during his TMS sessions one to two times weekly (online treatment). He also received one offline session weekly immediately before or after a TMS session. His treatment provider administered psychotherapy and managed the psychotropic medications. Various therapeutic modalities incorporated into sessions included behavioral activation and cognitive restructuring (a CBT approach), training using a progressive muscle relaxation exercise, and problem-focused therapy to assist with employment.

Practical implementation involved the selection of specific, effective therapeutic interventions. The components necessary to foster excellent therapeutic rapport included eye contact, positioning, volume of speech, and privacy. These were maintained by using various techniques. The provider sat directly in front of the patient at a comfortable height to maintain

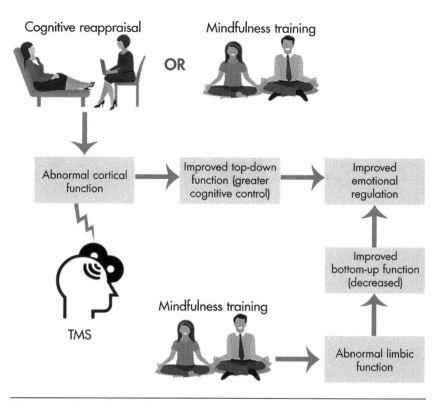

Figure 3–1. Effects of psychotherapy and transcranial magnetic stimulation (TMS) on neural networks.

Psychotherapy and TMS induce neuroplastic changes that normalize neural networks instrumental in mood regulation.

eye contact because the patient was in a fixed position during treatment. Both the provider and the patient were sensitive to the auditory interruptions of the TMS pulse trains. During the right-sided low-frequency treatment (1 pulse/second), each spoke at a slightly higher than average amplitude over the metronomic pulse delivery. Speech was paused (even mid-sentence) during the left-sided high-frequency treatment (10 pulses/second for 4 seconds) and then resumed during the intertrain interval (10 seconds). Ultimately, the patient achieved a 63% reduction in depressive symptoms as measured by the PHQ-9 and a 66% reduction in anxiety symptoms as measured by the Generalized Anxiety Disorder 7-item scale (GAD-7). In his final session, the patient reflected that the combination of psychotherapy and TMS was particularly helpful in identifying triggers and improving coping skills. In summary, practical barriers to implementing concurrent TMS and psychotherapy were quickly identified and adjusted to provide a successful online therapy course with TMS.

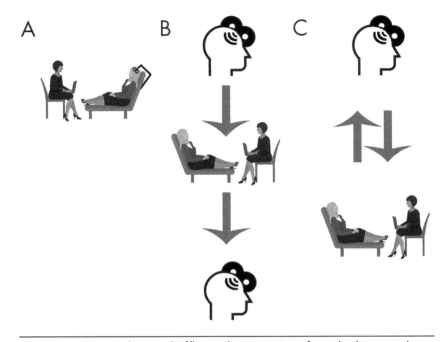

Figure 3–2. Online and offline administration of psychotherapy plus transcranial magnetic stimulation (TMS).

TMS and psychotherapy can be administered (**A**) during the same session (online), (**B**) sequentially, to prime one intervention (offline), or (**C**) randomly but during the same treatment course (offline).

Review of Literature

Donse et al. (2018) followed up a large cohort ($N=196$) of patients who received psychotherapy simultaneously during TMS sessions. Patients received at least 10 sessions of psychotherapy based on CBT principles administered during a TMS session by a psychotherapist. Patients found psychotherapy during TMS acceptable and completed an average of 20.9 (SD=7.5) sessions. Of the 196 patients starting treatment, 179 completed 10 sessions, 106 completed 20 sessions, 22 completed 30 sessions, 6 completed 40 sessions, and 3 completed 50 or more sessions. Sixty-six percent of patients responded, and 56% remitted. These results were better than those for previously published RCTs or outcome repository studies.

Brown University researchers tested two modified psychological protocols combined with TMS for MDD. In one pilot study, patients listened to mindfulness-based cognitive therapy audio tracks during sessions for

5 consecutive weeks beginning at week 2 of the TMS course (Cavallero et al. 2021). In addition, they received weekly support and education from the research staff. As a result, 56% of the eligible participants ($n=29$) consented to the study, and 19 completed it. Those who withdrew reported anxiety (3), loss of interest (1), dislike (1), falling asleep (1), and other (3). This response indicated a lack of feasibility in implementing mindfulness meditation during TMS stimulation. Those subjects who completed the meditation protocol with TMS reported significant reductions in depression ($P<0.01$) and perceived stress ($P<0.01$) and significantly enhanced quality of life ($P<0.01$) and aspects of mindfulness ($P<0.01$) (e.g., nonjudgment stance to inner experience and nonreactivity). Because the study was not blinded and had no control groups, conclusions are limited.

In another pilot study, 11 consecutive outpatients received a modified version of behavioral activation combined with TMS treatment (Russo et al. 2018). Before treatment, patients checked in and reviewed homework and goal attainment. After stimulation during the checkout process, patients confirmed new goals with staff. Patients who accepted modified behavioral activation within the usual 1-hour TMS appointments accomplished 77% of their therapeutic goals, improved across multiple domains of pleasure, and experienced reduced depression. Incorporating behavioral activation with TMS is feasible and may augment the effects of TMS.

In the largest RCT study, Duan et al. (2023) compared the synergistic effects of 4 weeks of TMS and 6 weeks of once-weekly group mindfulness-based stress reduction (MBSR) for poststroke depressed patients. Investigators allocated 72 patients equally to TMS plus MBSR, sham TMS plus MBSR, and sham TMS plus general psychological care. Researchers measured depression symptoms, cognition, sleep quality, and daily activities during and for 8 weeks after intervention. The repeated-measures analysis of variance showed a significant improvement in all variables in the TMS plus MBSR group compared with those receiving sham TMS plus MBSR ($P<0.05$) and sham TMS plus general psychological care ($P<0.05$). Pearson's correlation analysis indicated that improved depression correlated with improvements in cognition, activities of daily living, and sleep quality ($P<0.001$). The combined TMS plus MBSR treatment was effective in reducing depression and improving cognition, activities of daily living, and sleep. Because there was no TMS plus psychological care group in the study, however, it was unclear whether the combined intervention was better than TMS monotherapy. Table 3–2 lists key publications that combine TMS with psychotherapy online.

Evidence is emerging regarding the benefits of psychotherapy and TMS to treat a number of psychiatric disorders, including MDD. Research also

Table 3–2. Overview of psychotherapeutic modalities used with transcranial magnetic stimulation (TMS) for various disorders

Condition	Therapy	Delivery[a]	Key reference
Depression	Cognitive-behavioral therapy	Online	Vedeniapin et al. 2010
	Behavioral therapy	Online	Russo et al. 2018
	Mindfulness meditation	Online	Cavallero et al. 2021
PTSD	ERP	Online	Osuch et al. 2009
OCD	ERP	Offline	Grassi et al. 2015
	ERP	Online	Carmi et al. 2019
Smoking cessation	Exposure to cues with response prevention	Online	Zangen et al. 2021
Poststroke depression	Speech and language therapy	Offline	Yoon et al. 2015
	Virtual reality training	Online	Zheng et al. 2015
	Occupational therapy	Offline	Kakuda et al. 2010
Alzheimer's disease	Cognitive training	Offline	Rabey et al. 2013

Note. ERP=exposure and response prevention therapy.
[a]*Online* indicates therapy delivered simultaneously with TMS treatment. *Offline* indicates therapy delivered outside TMS treatment session but over the course of TMS treatment.

indicates that the effectiveness of TMS treatment depends on the baseline neural state of the subject. Thus, TMS may be more effective when applied to active rather than passive brain circuits, particularly for anxiety conditions and substance use disorders (Kearney-Ramos et al. 2019).

For example, Marin and Milad (2015) hypothesized that augmentation with TMS could facilitate the consolidation process of learning during exposure-based therapies and could improve responses for patients with treatment-resistant PTSD. In a crossover study, Osuch et al. (2009) randomly assigned nine adults with treatment-refractory PTSD to imaginal exposure therapy combined with 1-Hz TMS over the right dorsolateral prefrontal cortex (DLPFC) or a sham procedure. Before treatment, patients developed an individual exposure hierarchy consisting of 10 cues for use during their sessions. The list began with item 0, chosen by the subject as calming, with subsequent experiences eliciting incrementally increasing levels of distress. During the sessions, patients could control to what degree they were exposed to the traumatic experiences, talk about any traumatic cues, or remain silent.

All patients completed the 4-week protocol of imaginal exposure therapy during TMS (online therapy). Although overall effects were limited by the size of the study, active TMS treatment produced a large, although nonsignificant, effect on hyperarousal symptoms compared with sham TMS ($P<0.08$). Furthermore, 24-hour urinary norepinephrine and serum thyroxine levels increased, whereas prolactin levels decreased. The authors concluded that TMS plus imaginal exposure therapy was well tolerated and feasible and had symptomatic and physiological effects in patients with severe, treatment-refractory PTSD. Although these results are preliminary, they support conducting more extensive studies to clarify the effects of combining exposure therapy with TMS for PTSD.

In an individual case report, TMS enhanced the results of exposure and response prevention therapy for a patient with treatment-resistant OCD (Grassi et al. 2015). The participant in this report was a 32-year-old woman with severe OCD (since age 10 years) and concurrent mild depression who experienced low daily functioning. She did not respond to multiple serotonergic medications, augmentation with second-generation antipsychotics, and two different CBT trials at specialized OCD centers.

She then underwent 16 sessions of CBT, with the latter 10 centered on exposure and response prevention therapy exercises. Before each exposure session, she was given a high-frequency TMS session over the left DLPFC. A reduction of 32% from the Yale-Brown Obsessive Compulsive Scale (Y-BOCS) baseline score was observed after the final treatment session and was maintained at 6-, 12-, and 24-month follow-ups. She also reported a significantly improved quality of life and daily functioning. The authors concluded that TMS might enhance extinction learning because of its long-lasting effects on neuroplasticity, although further systematic studies are required to establish reliability.

This concept was further tested in a large randomized OCD study when subjects were first confronted with their obsessive triggers at the start of each TMS session. This confrontation was done so that the patients would have a Subjective Units of Distress Scale (SUDS) rating between 4 and 7 before the TMS treatment. A significant reduction in the Y-BOCS score was observed in patients who underwent active TMS treatment after exposure to their triggers compared with those who received a placebo. The response rates were 38.1% and 11.1%, respectively, demonstrating the effectiveness of TMS (Carmi et al. 2019).

A similar approach was used in a large prospective study on TMS for smoking cessation, in which subjects were presented with stimuli associated with smoking before each TMS or placebo session. The study found that quit rates were higher in the group that received active treatment plus exposure to smoking cues as early as 2 weeks into the study (Zangen et al. 2021; see also Chapter 7, "Transcranial Magnetic Stimulation for Disorders Other Than Depression").

In conclusion, for conditions such as PTSD, OCD, tobacco use disorder, and other substance use disorders, combining TMS with exposure and response prevention or cues that trigger cravings may be essential. This approach could enhance the neuroplastic changes needed to support long-term cognitive-affective and behavioral modifications in these conditions.

Combining Therapy, Behavioral Skills, and Exercise With TMS

Several depression-specific therapies and behavioral skills can be combined with TMS during and outside of treatment sessions (Society of Clinical Psychology 2022). As highlighted in the "Rationale for Combining TMS and Psychotherapy" section, therapy received outside treatment sessions is called an offline intervention. In contrast, modalities administered during the TMS therapy session are online interventions. Behavioral activation, cognitive therapy, and interpersonal psychotherapy have firm research support as monotherapies for patients with depression. These treatments are used in clinical practice and should be considered optimal modalities to combine with TMS for patients with TRD. Before therapy is initiated, it is essential to understand the patient's history of therapy because it helps stage their level of treatment resistance and provides an in-

Table 3–3. Offline therapeutic activities to augment antidepressant effects of transcranial magnetic stimulation

Walking at least 30 minutes/day
Doing yoga
Practicing meditation
Hiking
Playing tennis and other sports
Engaging in hobbies such as knitting
Practicing good sleep hygiene
Healthy eating (e.g., reduction or elimination of sugar or gluten)
Joining a jogging or running group
Reestablishing friendships
Journaling
Moderating caffeine and alcohol intake
Increasing exposure to natural light
Volunteering or community service
Observing religious and/or spiritual activities

ventory of previous therapies. Records should document the approximate start and stop dates of treatment, frequency of sessions, type of psychotherapy or skills taught, focus of the treatment, and degree and name of the therapist. If validated instruments were used to measure the change in depressive symptoms, then pre- and posttreatment scores should be documented. Patients can usually report a subjective sense of whether the treatment was helpful, partially helpful, or unhelpful. Some patients hesitate to restart or continue therapy with TMS because they may perceive that TMS therapy did not work or have concerns about time constraints as a barrier to pursuing both treatments. Building motivation, establishing goals, and exploring negative perceptions about therapy are instrumental for patients to succeed when combining TMS with psychotherapy.

Engaging in healthy behaviors and activities between TMS treatment sessions can benefit patients. Table 3–3 lists multiple activities, such as exercise, yoga, and journaling, that can assist patients in countering the symptomatic isolation and withdrawal of severe depression. Patients can be encouraged by their TMS clinician and technician to engage in such activities throughout a TMS course. Anecdotally, patients who engage in healthy behaviors have more significant and durable symptom reductions.

Many brief psychotherapeutic skills can be taught or reinforced by the TMS technician during treatment sessions (Table 3–4). For example, negative thinking about oneself, others, and one's future (Beck's negative

Table 3–4. Brief online therapeutic activities for use during
             transcranial magnetic stimulation therapy sessions

Goal setting

Performing positive imagery exercise

Completing body scan meditation

Practicing mindful breathing

Doing progressive muscle relaxation

Acquiring psychoeducation about depression

Creating a sleep diary

Creating a nutrition diary

Using breathing retraining to cope with anxiety

Identifying automatic thoughts and cognitive errors

Modifying negative thinking

Identifying triggers for depression

Scheduling activities

Obtaining psychoeducation regarding sleep

Increasing psychoeducation regarding exercise

Creating symptom diaries

Engaging in leisure activities (listening to music or a podcast, watching
television)

triad; Beck et al. 1987) is pervasive in depression. Learning to identify the
triggers for negative thinking, maladaptive thought patterns, and typical
cognitive errors can be accomplished with basic training and TMS technician reinforcement. Acquisition of this type of skill is a neurobehavioral
intervention with a specific functional effect on the DLPFC, which correlates with improved functioning and *top-down* control of the limbic system (Ritchey et al. 2011).

Conclusion

Research supporting the combination of TMS with pharmacotherapy and
psychotherapy is still evolving. In light of that, the available preclinical
and clinical data to guide decisions about combining or sequencing TMS
with pharmacotherapy should be considered preliminary. In a naturalistic
setting, however, combining TMS with other effective treatments may
help patients recover fully. For example, although investigational at this

time, TMS augmentation strategies, such as adding D-cycloserine or psychostimulants and reducing or eliminating benzodiazepines, may represent viable strategies to manage more resistant depression and hasten the onset of efficacy.

A patient's brain state during TMS stimulation matters. Supporting treatment sessions with online therapeutic interventions and adjusting medications before a patient starts TMS optimize the patient's brain state and may enhance outcomes. How patients manage their experiences with psychotherapy and medications between TMS treatments (offline) also may assist with improvements. Improved medication adherence and engagement in healthy activities and behaviors can improve the overall outcome. Thus, assessing a patient's pharmacotherapy and psychotherapy history and optimally integrating these treatments with TMS are essential to managing the whole patient and increasing long-term remission rates.

KEY POINTS

- The role of transcranial magnetic stimulation (TMS) augmentation strategies is supported by large acute studies and maintenance studies conducted under naturalistic conditions.

- Because most patients in clinical practice receive psychotropic medications plus TMS, heightened awareness of potential changes in efficacy and risks is required.

- The prescription of medications with TMS requires the psychopharmacotherapist and TMS clinician to communicate clearly and clarify the roles and responsibilities of each.

- Patients receiving TMS for depression should be encouraged to engage in therapies delivered offline. These include cognitive-behavioral therapy, behavioral activation, mindfulness-based cognitive-behavioral therapy, and interpersonal therapy.

- TMS technicians with appropriate supervision and training can provide support for brief therapeutic activities that do not require a licensed clinician and can offer options to integrate mindfulness or cognitive-behavioral therapy exercises during the patient's treatment.

- Patients should be encouraged to engage in healthy behaviors, lifestyles, and relationships while receiving TMS to achieve the best chance of recovery.

References

Bajbouj M, Padberg F: A perfect match: noninvasive brain stimulation and psychotherapy. Eur Arch Psychiatry Clin Neurosci 264(1)(Suppl 1):S27–S33, 2014 25253645

Beck AT, Rush AJ, Shaw BF, et al: Cognitive Therapy of Depression. New York, Guilford, 1987

Berlim MT, Van den Eynde F, Daskalakis ZJ: High-frequency repetitive transcranial magnetic stimulation accelerates and enhances the clinical response to antidepressants in major depression: a meta-analysis of randomized, double-blind, and sham-controlled trials. J Clin Psychiatry 74(2):e122–e129, 2013 23473357

Berlim MT, Van den Eynde F, Tovar-Perdomo S, et al: Augmenting antidepressants with deep transcranial magnetic stimulation (DTMS) in treatment-resistant major depression. World J Biol Psychiatry 15(7):570–578, 2014 25050453

Best SRD, Pavel DG, Haustrup N: Combination therapy with transcranial magnetic stimulation and ketamine for treatment-resistant depression: a long-term retrospective review of clinical use. Heliyon 5(8):e02187, 2019 31440588

Blumberger DM, Vila-Rodriguez F, Thorpe KE, et al: Effectiveness of theta burst versus high-frequency repetitive transcranial magnetic stimulation in patients with depression (THREE-D): a randomised non-inferiority trial. Lancet 391(10131):1683–1692, 2018 29726344

Brown JC, Higgins ES, George MS: Synaptic plasticity 101: the story of the AMPA receptor for the brain stimulation practitioner. Neuromodulation 25(8):1289–1298, 2022 35088731

Carmi L, Tendler A, Bystritsky A, et al: Efficacy and safety of deep transcranial magnetic stimulation for obsessive-compulsive disorder: a prospective multicenter randomized, double-blind placebo-controlled trial. Am J Psychiatry 176(11):931–938, 2019 31109199

Carpenter LL, Janicak PG, Aaronson ST, et al: Transcranial magnetic stimulation (TMS) for major depression: a multisite, naturalistic, observational study of acute treatment outcomes in clinical practice. Depress Anxiety 29(7):587–596, 2012 22689344

Cavallero F, Gold MC, Tirrell E, et al: Audio-guided mindfulness meditation during transcranial magnetic stimulation sessions for the treatment of major depressive disorder: a pilot feasibility study. Front Psychol 12:678911, 2021 34484035

Chiesa A, Serretti A, Jakobsen JC: Mindfulness: top-down or bottom-up emotion regulation strategy? Clin Psychol Rev 33(1):82–96, 2013 23142788

Cole J, Sohn MN, Harris AD, et al: Efficacy of adjunctive d-cycloserine to intermittent theta-burst stimulation for major depressive disorder: a randomized clinical trial. JAMA Psychiatry 79(12):1153–1161, 2022 36223114

Conca A, Koppi S, König P, et al: Transcranial magnetic stimulation: a novel antidepressive strategy? Neuropsychobiology 34(4):204–207, 1996 9121622

Conca A, Swoboda E, König P, et al: Clinical impacts of single transcranial magnetic stimulation (sTMS) as an add-on therapy in severely depressed patients under SSRI treatment. Hum Psychopharmacol 15(6):429–438, 2000 12404305

Deppe M, Abdelnaim M, Hebel T, et al: Concomitant lorazepam use and antidepressive efficacy of repetitive transcranial magnetic stimulation in a naturalistic setting. Eur Arch Psychiatry Clin Neurosci 271(1):61–67, 2021 32648109

Dobek CE, Blumberger DM, Downar J, et al: Risk of seizures in transcranial magnetic stimulation: a clinical review to inform consent process focused on bupropion. Neuropsychiatr Dis Treat 11:2975–2987, 2015 26664122

Donse L, Padberg F, Sack AT, et al: Simultaneous rTMS and psychotherapy in major depressive disorder: clinical outcomes and predictors from a large naturalistic study. Brain Stimul 11(2):337–345, 2018 29174304

Duan H, Yan X, Meng S, et al: Effectiveness evaluation of repetitive transcranial magnetic stimulation therapy combined with mindfulness-based stress reduction for people with post-stroke depression: a randomized controlled trial. Int J Environ Res Public Health 20(2):930, 2023 36673684

Dunner DL, Aaronson ST, Sackeim HA, et al: A multisite, naturalistic, observational study of transcranial magnetic stimulation for patients with pharmacoresistant major depressive disorder: durability of benefit over a 1-year follow-up period. J Clin Psychiatry 75(12):1394–1401, 2014 25271871

Elkrief L, Payette O, Foucault JN, et al: Transcranial magnetic stimulation and intravenous ketamine combination therapy for treatment-resistant bipolar depression: a case report. Front Psychiatry 13:986378, 2022 36213934

Fitzgerald PB, Daskalakis ZJ, Hoy KE: Benzodiazepine use and response to repetitive transcranial magnetic stimulation in major depressive disorder. Brain Stimul 13(3):694–695, 2020 32289699

Gersner R, Kravetz E, Feil J, et al: Long-term effects of repetitive transcranial magnetic stimulation on markers for neuroplasticity: differential outcomes in anesthetized and awake animals. J Neurosci 31(20):7521–7526, 2011 21593336

Grassi G, Godini L, Grippo A, et al: Enhancing cognitive-behavioral therapy with repetitive transcranial magnetic stimulation in refractory obsessive-compulsive-disorder: a case report. Brain Stimul 8(1):160–161, 2015 25456982

Harada T, Sakamoto K, Ishigooka J: Incidence and predictors of activation syndrome induced by antidepressants. Depress Anxiety 25(12):1014–1019, 2008 18781664

Harel EV, Zangen A, Roth Y, et al: H-coil repetitive transcranial magnetic stimulation for the treatment of bipolar depression: an add-on, safety and feasibility study. World J Biol Psychiatry 12(2):119–126, 2011 20854181

Hunter AM, Minzenberg MJ, Cook IA, et al: Concomitant medication use and clinical outcome of repetitive transcranial magnetic stimulation (rTMS) treatment of major depressive disorder. Brain Behav 9(5):e01275, 2019 30941915

Isserles M, Rosenberg O, Dannon P, et al: Cognitive-emotional reactivation during deep transcranial magnetic stimulation over the prefrontal cortex of depressive patients affects antidepressant outcome. J Affect Disord 128(3):235–242, 2011 20663568

Janicak PG, O'Reardon JP, Sampson SM, et al: Transcranial magnetic stimulation in the treatment of major depressive disorder: a comprehensive summary of safety experience from acute exposure, extended exposure, and during reintroduction treatment. J Clin Psychiatry 69(2):222–232, 2008 18232722

Janicak PG, Nahas Z, Lisanby SH, et al: Durability of clinical benefit with transcranial magnetic stimulation (TMS) in the treatment of pharmacoresistant major depression: assessment of relapse during a 6-month, multisite, open-label study. Brain Stimul 3(4):187–199, 2010 20965447

Kakuda W, Abo M, Kaito N, et al: Six-day course of repetitive transcranial magnetic stimulation plus occupational therapy for post-stroke patients with upper limb hemiparesis: a case series study. Disabil Rehabil 32(10):801–807, 2010 20367405

Kaster TS, Downar J, Vila-Rodriguez F, et al: Trajectories of response to dorsolateral prefrontal rTMS in major depression: a THREE-D study. Am J Psychiatry 176(5):367–375, 2019 30764649

Kearney-Ramos TE, Dowdle LT, Mithoefer OJ, et al: State-dependent effects of ventromedial prefrontal cortex continuous thetaburst stimulation on cocaine cue reactivity in chronic cocaine users. Front Psychiatry 10:317, 2019 31133897

Korchounov A, Ziemann U: Neuromodulatory neurotransmitters influence LTP-like plasticity in human cortex: a pharmaco-TMS study. Neuropsychopharmacology 36(9):1894–1902, 2011 21544070

Lerner AJ, Wassermann EM, Tamir DI: Seizures from transcranial magnetic stimulation 2012–2016: results of a survey of active laboratories and clinics. Clin Neurophysiol 130(8):1409–1416, 2019 31104898

Li X, Tenebäck CC, Nahas Z, et al: Interleaved transcranial magnetic stimulation/functional MRI confirms that lamotrigine inhibits cortical excitability in healthy young men. Neuropsychopharmacology 29(7):1395–1407, 2004 15100699

Liu B, Zhang Y, Zhang L, et al: Repetitive transcranial magnetic stimulation as an augmentative strategy for treatment-resistant depression, a meta-analysis of randomized, double-blind and sham-controlled study. BMC Psychiatry 14:342, 2014 25433539

Mantovani A, Pavlicova M, Avery D, et al: Long-term efficacy of repeated daily prefrontal transcranial magnetic stimulation (TMS) in treatment-resistant depression. Depress Anxiety 29(10):883–890, 2012 22689290

Marin M, Milad MR: Neuromodulation approaches for the treatment of post-traumatic stress disorder: stimulating the brain following exposure-based therapy. Curr Behav Neurosci Rep 2(2):67–71, 2015

Mojtabai R, Olfson M: National trends in mental health care for US adolescents. JAMA Psychiatry 77(7):703–714, 2020 32211824

Mufti MA, Holtzheimer PE III, Epstein CM, et al: Bupropion decreases resting motor threshold: a case report. Brain Stimul 3(3):177–180, 2010 20633447

O'Reardon JP, Solvason HB, Janicak PG, et al: Efficacy and safety of transcranial magnetic stimulation in the acute treatment of major depression: a multisite randomized controlled trial. Biol Psychiatry 62(11):1208–1216, 2007 17573044

Osuch EA, Benson BE, Luckenbaugh DA, et al: Repetitive TMS combined with exposure therapy for PTSD: a preliminary study. J Anxiety Disord 23(1):54–59, 2009 18455908

Papakostas GI, Trivedi MH, Shelton RC, et al: Comparative effectiveness research trial for antidepressant incomplete and non-responders with treatment resistant depression (ASCERTAIN-TRD): a randomized clinical trial. Mol Psychiatry 2024

Perera T, George MS, Grammer G, et al: The Clinical TMS Society consensus review and treatment recommendations for TMS therapy for major depressive disorder. Brain Stimul 9(3):336–346, 2016 27090022

Philip NS, Carpenter SL, Ridout SJ, et al: 5Hz repetitive transcranial magnetic stimulation to left prefrontal cortex for major depression. J Affect Disord 186:13–17, 2015 26210705

Rabey JM, Dobronevsky E, Aichenbaum S, et al: Repetitive transcranial magnetic stimulation combined with cognitive training is a safe and effective modality for the treatment of Alzheimer's disease: a randomized, double-blind study. J Neural Transm (Vienna) 120(5):813–819, 2013 23076723

Ritchey M, Dolcos F, Eddington KM, et al: Neural correlates of emotional processing in depression: changes with cognitive behavioral therapy and predictors of treatment response. J Psychiatr Res 45(5):577–587, 2011 20934190

Rossi S, Hallett M, Rossini PM, et al: Safety, ethical considerations, and application guidelines for the use of transcranial magnetic stimulation in clinical practice and research. Clin Neurophysiol 120(12):2008–2039, 2009 19833552

Rossi S, Antal A, Bestmann S, et al: Safety and recommendations for TMS use in healthy subjects and patient populations, with updates on training, ethical and regulatory issues: expert guidelines. Clin Neurophysiol 132(1):269–306, 2021 33243615

Russo GB, Tirrell E, Busch A, et al: Behavioral activation therapy during transcranial magnetic stimulation for major depressive disorder. J Affect Disord 236:101–104, 2018 29723763

Sackeim HA: The definition and meaning of treatment-resistant depression. J Clin Psychiatry 62(Suppl 16):10–17, 2001 11480879

Sheline Y, Shou H, Yang Z, et al: Cognitive behavioral therapy improves frontoparietal network neuroplasticity across major depression and PTSD: evidence from longitudinal fMRI studies of functional connectivity. Biol Psychiatry 81(10):S143–S144, 2017

Siddiqi SH, Kording KP, Parvizi J, et al: Causal mapping of human brain function. Nat Rev Neurosci 23(6):361–375, 2022 35444305

Silvanto J, Muggleton N, Walsh V: State-dependency in brain stimulation studies of perception and cognition. Trends Cogn Sci 12(12):447–454, 2008 18951833

Silvanto J, Bona S, Marelli M, et al: On the mechanisms of transcranial magnetic stimulation (TMS): how brain state and baseline performance level determine behavioral effects of TMS. Front Psychol 9:741, 2018 29867693

Society of Clinical Psychology: Depression. Atlanta, GA, Division 12, American Psychological Association, 2022. Available at: http://www.div12.org/psychological-treatments/disorders/depression. Accessed September 22, 2024.

Su TP, Huang CC, Wei IH: Add-on rTMS for medication-resistant depression: a randomized, double-blind, sham-controlled trial in Chinese patients. J Clin Psychiatry 66(7):930–937, 2005 16013911

Tang YY, Hölzel BK, Posner MI: The neuroscience of mindfulness meditation. Nat Rev Neurosci 16(4):213–225, 2015 25783612

Vedeniapin A, Cheng L, George MS: Feasibility of simultaneous cognitive behavioral therapy and left prefrontal rTMS for treatment resistant depression. Brain Stimul 3(4):207–210, 2010 20965449

Wilke SA, Johnson CL, Corlier J, et al: Psychostimulant use and clinical outcome of repetitive transcranial magnetic stimulation treatment of major depressive disorder. Depress Anxiety 39(5):397–406, 2022 35389536

Yoon TH, Han SJ, Yoon TS, et al: Therapeutic effect of repetitive magnetic stimulation combined with speech and language therapy in post-stroke non-fluent aphasia. NeuroRehabilitation 36(1):107–114, 2015 25547773

Zangen A, Moshe H, Martinez D, et al: Repetitive transcranial magnetic stimulation for smoking cessation: a pivotal multicenter double-blind randomized controlled trial. World Psychiatry 20(3):397–404, 2021 34505368

Zheng CJ, Liao WJ, Xia WG: Effect of combined low-frequency repetitive transcranial magnetic stimulation and virtual reality training on upper limb function in subacute stroke: a double-blind randomized controlled trail. J Huazhong Univ Sci Technolog Med Sci 35(2):248–254, 2015 25877360

Ziemann U: Pharmaco-transcranial magnetic stimulation studies of motor excitability. Handb Clin Neurol 116:387–397, 2013 24112911

4

Transcranial Magnetic Stimulation for the Treatment of Other Mood Disorders

Juan F. Garzon, M.D.
Scott T. Aaronson, M.D.
Paul E. Croarkin, D.O., M.S.

In 2008, the FDA cleared repetitive transcranial magnetic stimulation (TMS) for treatment of major depressive disorder (MDD) in adults who did not receive benefit from antidepressant medications. Additional research and clinical practice confirmed the safety and efficacy of TMS in MDD (see Chapter 2, "Transcranial Magnetic Stimulation Therapy for Major Depression"), and clinicians and researchers rapidly began exploring the utility of TMS for other populations. Early work suggested that this noninvasive form of brain stimulation may benefit other disorders, such as bipolar depression, perinatal depression, adolescent depression, and late-life depression (LLD), thereby offering new options to additional psychiatric populations with limited effective therapeutics.

Bipolar depression is distinct from unipolar depression in its pathophysiology; it presents a significant disease burden and lacks sufficient evidence to guide clinical treatment. Furthermore, recent medication development efforts for bipolar depression have concentrated on second-generation antipsychotics, which have an unacceptable side-effect burden for long-term use. *Perinatal depression* is a common and impairing condition that unfortunately is often undertreated. *Adolescent depression* is a global public health problem contributing to academic failure, delays in social development, substance use, teenage pregnancy, and death from suicide. Current treatment options for adolescent depression, which rely primarily on selective serotonin reuptake inhibitors (SSRIs) and evidence-based psychotherapeutic approaches such as cognitive-behavioral therapy (CBT), are often ineffective. *LLD* is frequently undiagnosed; however, even when properly identified and treated, it follows a more insidious course than depression in younger populations.

In this chapter, we survey recent research and clinical experience focused on the use of TMS in bipolar depression, perinatal depression, adolescent depression, and LLD. Although existing information is nascent and more extensive randomized controlled trials (RCTs) are underway, initial experience suggests that TMS may be a safe and effective alternative treatment for these indications. Unique risk factors (e.g., the potential induction of mania and unknown, untoward effects on neurodevelopment) must be carefully considered, but the consequences of untreated or inadequately treated depression in bipolar disorder, during the perinatal period, in adolescence, and later in life are significant. Existing knowledge may inform clinicians considering the off-label use of TMS in these populations.

Bipolar Depression

Current Treatment Paradigm

Within the scope of mood disorders, bipolar depression is especially difficult to manage. Treatment practice typically uses antidepressants combined with mood-stabilizing agents, despite the absence of clear evidence supporting the efficacy of such treatment. Findings from the National Institute of Mental Health–funded Systematic Treatment Enhancement Program for Bipolar Disorder (STEP-BD), a large study that sought to identify best treatment practices in bipolar disorder, supported the notion that antidepressants added to mood stabilizers do not improve outcomes and may even carry the risk of precipitating a mixed or manic episode (El-Mallakh et al. 2015).

The current FDA-approved evidence base for the treatment of bipolar depression is limited to certain second-generation antipsychotics, one of which is paired with an SSRI (i.e., quetiapine, lurasidone, cariprazine, lumateperone, or olanzapine plus fluoxetine) (Levenberg and Cordner 2022). The high side-effect burden (especially weight gain, sedation, and metabolic syndrome) of these agents makes them an unacceptable choice for many patients. One of the challenges in developing safe and effective treatments for bipolar depression is that this population is quite heterogeneous, with subgroups that may require different pharmacological interventions (Levenberg and Cordner 2022; Mendlewicz et al. 2010). Treatment-resistant bipolar depression in which patients do not obtain sustained symptomatic remission for 8 consecutive weeks after two different trials of the recommended treatments is documented in about one-third of patients with bipolar disorder (Mendlewicz et al. 2010).

Another challenge with the use of antidepressants is that it is hard, if not impossible, to target only one pole of a cyclical disorder with medications affecting nerve cells and receptor sites over extended periods. For patients with rapid-cycling bipolar disorder, continued use of antidepressants is associated with worse outcomes (El-Mallakh et al. 2015). This raises the question of whether neurostimulation such as TMS can provide briefer, episode-based interventions for bipolar depression without the risk of manic switches or mood destabilization.

Evidence Base for TMS in Bipolar Depression: Randomized Sham-Controlled Trials and Meta-Analyses

Given the substantial unmet needs of patients with bipolar depression, a therapeutic TMS treatment has appeal. Conceptually, TMS treatments for bipolar depression may target dysregulated prefrontal and subcortical neurocircuitry, where excitatory and inhibitory imbalances are implicated in affect, neurocognition, and psychomotor retardation. Previous work has implicated the salience, sensorimotor, default mode, and central executive networks in pathophysiology that may be treatment targets for TMS (Bi et al. 2022). Although interest in using TMS to treat bipolar depression extends back two decades, the heterogeneity of study designs hampers the development of a clear evidence base. Studies have examined continuous, intermittent, unilateral, and bilateral modes at different stimulation frequencies (i.e., 1 Hz, 5 Hz, 10 Hz, and 50 Hz) over the dorsolateral prefrontal cortex (DLPFC), with durations between 1 and 4 weeks (McGirr et al. 2021; Nguyen et al. 2021; Tee and Au 2020).

Two recent meta-analyses of RCTs for TMS in bipolar depression found superior responses for treatment compared with placebo (Nguyen et al. 2021; Tee and Au 2020). However, only high-frequency TMS over the left DLPFC showed statistical superiority, whereas bilateral stimulation and low-frequency TMS did not (Nguyen et al. 2021). Otherwise, the low rates of mood switching with TMS are encouraging. Six RCTs that documented TMS side effects did not report serious events, noting only a hypomanic switch after 3 weeks of TMS (10 Hz) over the left DLPFC that resolved spontaneously within hours (Tee and Au 2020).

A recent crossover sham-controlled trial found greater changes in depressive symptoms for participants receiving TMS. In this study, 1,000 pulses were delivered twice daily over the left DLPFC for 2 weeks (10-Hz, 4-second trains with 20-second intertrain intervals) (Zengin et al. 2022).

However, trials with theta burst stimulation (TBS) (triplet bursts at 50 Hz repeated at 5 Hz for 2 seconds) found less benefit among this population. In one trial that was discontinued after a futility analysis, participants received intermittent TBS (iTBS) or sham interventions (with 8-second intertrain intervals) over the left DLPFC for 4 weeks. The response rate was 16.7% for patients assigned to active iTBS and 15.8% for the sham group (McGirr et al. 2021). Another recent pilot study examined continuous TBS targeting the right DLPFC in 19 participants for 5 days (three daily sessions of 600 pulses). This study was likely underpowered but did not show efficacy of iTBS in acute-phase bipolar depression (Mallik et al. 2023).

In summary, the existing evidence base is heterogeneous for treatment delivery, type of bipolar disorder (i.e., I or II), and use of concomitant medication (subjects were generally not taking antidepressants but could take mood stabilizers depending on the study). However, the trend is to favor unilateral, left-sided high-frequency treatment over intermittent, right-sided, or sequential bilateral stimulations for bipolar depression. However, no head-to-head trials are available to guide clinicians on the optimal stimulation protocol. Thus, an ongoing need remains for rigorous, adequately powered RCTs of TMS for bipolar depression (Nguyen et al. 2021; Tee and Au 2020).

Clinical Experience With TMS in Bipolar Depression: Open-Label Trials and Case Reviews

Clinicians providing TMS to patients for bipolar depression report varied results, in part because of population heterogeneity and varying treatment parameters. A summary of the larger cohorts (with more than 15 patients) is provided in Table 4–1.

A retrospective study evaluating the DLPFC TMS response of 248 patients with unipolar ($n=102$) and bipolar ($n=146$) depressive disorders did not find a significant difference in the effect of the depression type on

Table 4–1. Open-label transcranial magnetic stimulation studies in bipolar depression (N>15)

Reference	N	Treatment location; coil type	Frequency; intensity; pulses/day	Sessions	Outcomes; measurement	Side effects
Harel et al. 2011	19	L-DLPFC; H coil	20 Hz; 120% MT; 1,680 pulses	20 over 4 weeks	52.6% response, 63.2% remission; HDRS	No mania or hypomania, one generalized seizure
Connolly et al. 2012	20	L-DLPFC; figure-eight coil	10 Hz; 120% MT; 3,000 pulses	30 over 6 weeks	35% response, 15% remission; CGI	No serious adverse events
Goldwaser et al. 2020	39	L-DLPFC; figure-eight coil	10 Hz; 120% MT; 3,000 pulses	Up to 30 over 6 weeks	BP1: 44% response, 72% remission BP2: 67% response, 28% remission; MADRS	Treatment-emergent agitation in 17% of BP1 and 5% of BP2, no mania or hypomania
Koutsomitros et al. 2022	23	L-DLPFC; figure-eight coil	10 Hz; 120% MT; 1,000 pulses	20 over 4 weeks	61% remission after 20th session, 78% remission 1-month follow-up; BDI	No serious adverse events, but one patient dropped out because of irritability

Note. BDI=Beck Depression Inventory; BP1=patients with bipolar I disorder; BP2=patients with bipolar II disorder; CGI=Clinical Global Impression Scale; HDRS=Hamilton Depression Rating Scale; L-DLPFC=left dorsolateral prefrontal cortex; MADRS=Montgomery-Åsberg Depression Rating Scale; MT=motor threshold.

treatment response. Only age and cognitive-affective symptoms were significant predictors of TMS response. Cognitive-affective symptom predominance and young age were associated with a higher benefit in both forms of depression (Rostami et al. 2017).

A retrospective study of 100 consecutive patients treated for depression in a university-based TMS clinic (Connolly et al. 2012) reported a 35% response rate and a 15% remission rate in 20 patients with bipolar depression treated for 6 weeks with adjunctive TMS. The treatment was well tolerated, and there were no reports of manic symptoms, but the overall response and remission rates were lower in this subgroup compared with the patients with major depression.

A retrospective analysis of 39 patients with bipolar I or II depression treated at a specialized hospital-based TMS clinic (Goldwaser et al. 2020) found higher response rates in the bipolar group than in the unipolar group. All patients were treated with left-sided high-frequency stimulation at 10 Hz, the standard protocol for major depression. Every patient took at least one mood stabilizer, and four patients with bipolar II disorder continued taking antidepressant medication. All patients had experienced at least two and up to six adequate medication trial failures for their depressive episodes. For the patients with bipolar I disorder, the response rate was 72% (13/18), and the remission rate was 44% (8/18). For the patients with bipolar II disorder, the response rate was 67% (14/21), and the remission rate was 28% (5/18). In the context of these favorable response and remission rates, the authors speculated that bipolar depression may be a narrow phenotype for TMS intervention compared with unipolar depression. These data are shown in Figure 4–1.

Agitation leading to discontinuation was seen in 17% (3/18) of the bipolar I group and 5% (1/21) of the bipolar II group. The agitation occurred within the first 2 weeks of treatment and did not meet criteria for mania or hypomania. Among those achieving remission, the average number of treatments to remission was 22. Compared with 175 patients with unipolar depression treated at the same center, the patients with bipolar disorder had a higher average remission rate (36% vs. 31%), higher response rate (69% vs. 62%), and shorter course to remission (i.e., 22 vs. 29 sessions). Other than agitation, no significant adverse events occurred.

Open Questions

The clinical use of TMS for bipolar depression has outpaced the creation of a clear evidence base to support the safest and most effective use of this intervention. This population has substantial unmet clinical needs. TMS may, indeed, offer a nonpharmacological treatment option that can be

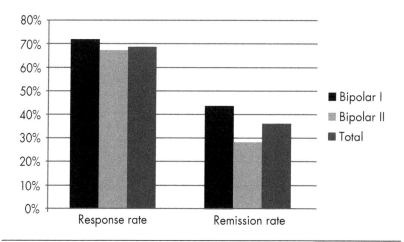

Figure 4–1. Transcranial magnetic stimulation response and remission rates in patients with bipolar I and II depression.

Source. Adapted from Goldwaser et al. 2020.

used episodically for depressive mood episodes, with a remarkably benign side-effect profile compared with systemically administered medications.

However, some questions remain:

- What is the optimal stimulation protocol (e.g., treatment duration, frequency, and magnetic coil positioning) for patients with bipolar depression?
- Should different treatment parameters (e.g., length of session, course of treatment, and 5- vs. 8- vs. 10-Hz stimulation frequency) be used for bipolar depression than for unipolar depression?
- Should TMS be administered with medications?
- Should treatment be given with or without mood stabilizers?
- Is TMS less or more effective when delivered with concurrent anticonvulsants used to treat bipolar disorders?
- Should patients stop taking antidepressants before TMS is initiated?
- Should patients with bipolar I disorder and bipolar II disorder receive different treatments?

Treatment Considerations and Recommendations

Table 4–2 lists treatment considerations and recommendations that were extrapolated from the existing evidence and clinical experience with the management of bipolar disorder and from the TMS treatment of unipolar depression.

Table 4–2. Treatment considerations and recommendations for transcranial magnetic stimulation (TMS) in bipolar depression

Establish a clear diagnosis with regard to the phase of the bipolar illness. Patients with bipolar I disorder are at higher risk for mixed or manic switches than are patients with bipolar II disorder and may need more protection with mood stabilizer support. Generally, patients in the mixed or manic phase of bipolar disorder are not good candidates for TMS, and no evidence supports its use. It is also doubtful that TMS can alleviate associated psychotic symptoms.

Optimize mood stabilizer prior to initiating TMS. The history of each patient's illness should help guide clinical decisions. Patients with higher risk of rapid or complex cycling or greater intensity of mania may do better with lithium or valproate plus a second-generation antipsychotic. Patients with a low risk of instability may be managed with lamotrigine. Patients should take a mood stabilizer for a minimum of 2 weeks before starting TMS.

Remember that antidepressants may be problematic. No clear evidence supports the use of antidepressants in this population. Give the patient at least 1–2 weeks to taper off antidepressants.

Evaluate patients with bipolar disorder at least weekly while they are receiving TMS. This population is at higher risk for manic switches and is more likely to see earlier response and remission. Furthermore, these patients are at risk for premature discontinuation of TMS secondary to treatment-emergent agitation. Consider using the Young Mania Rating Scale (YMRS) and the Generalized Anxiety Disorder 7-item scale (GAD-7) to monitor for treatment-emergent agitation or subsyndromal manic symptoms. Use a depression rating scale such as the Montgomery-Åsberg Depression Rating Scale (MADRS) to determine severity of illness, and consider stopping TMS if remission criteria are met or if improvement has plateaued for 2 weeks after at least 25 treatments.

Keep in mind that treatment parameters do not have a clear evidence base. Meta-analyses supported benefit for left-sided high-frequency treatment, but the evidence to justify right-sided and sequential bilateral treatment is less clear (Mallik et al. 2023; Nguyen et al. 2021). Most TMS centers use the same parameters for bipolar depression as for unipolar depression, that is, high-frequency stimulation in the left dorsolateral prefrontal cortex.

Collect data and measure symptom improvement with both patient questionnaires and validated clinician rating scales. The more extensive the clinical experience is, the more information can be gathered to optimize treatment with TMS in patients with bipolar depression.

Clinical Vignette 1

A 40-year-old single woman who is a successful entrepreneur has been depressed for the past 6 months and has been mostly housebound because of her symptoms. Trials of several antidepressants from different classes were unsuccessful because of the lack of response at adequate dosage and duration or intolerable agitation and insomnia. Her initial diagnosis was unipolar depression, but consultation indicated a long history of psychomotor agitation, decreased need for sleep, and frequent racing thoughts. One parent also had a history of bipolar disorder. Subsequent interviews elicited that the patient has a complex pattern of cycling in her work: she is unable to function for months at a time but then has weeks of extreme productivity, somewhat marred by pressure of speech, a brusque interpersonal style, the ability to function on 2 hours of sleep, and a sharp increase in alcohol consumption. Her diagnosis was changed to bipolar I disorder, and she began taking lithium.

After 4 weeks with an adequate blood level of the medication, the patient's depression persisted, and she was recommended for a trial of TMS, which was administered over the left DLPFC at 10 Hz. She experienced a significant improvement in mood after 1 week and full remission after 15 sessions, without manic activation. Acute TMS treatment was then tapered. She had minor recurrences of her depression when she returned to work, but she responded to one TMS session every 2 weeks to successfully maintain remission.

Perinatal Depression

Perinatal (prenatal and postpartum) depression is a common disabling condition that is underdiagnosed and undertreated. Treatment is often suboptimal, with the potential for substantial untoward effects on mothers, fetuses, and developing neonates. For example, depression during the perinatal period is associated with problematic lifestyle choices such as nicotine and alcohol use, substandard self-care, and considerable risk for death from suicide. These factors may present long-term negative consequences for child development given that exposure to maternal depression can create physiological and psychological stressors for the fetus or infant. These adverse effects affect placental epigenetic changes, fetal brain development, language development, and mother-infant bonding. Offspring of depressed mothers have an increased risk for depression, anxiety, and functional impairment (Kim et al. 2015; Susser et al. 2016).

Treatment of perinatal depression typically involves evidence-based psychotherapeutic approaches such as CBT, interpersonal psychotherapy, pharmacotherapy with SSRIs, or the combination of psychotherapy and antidepressants; brexanolone can be prescribed for postpartum depression. The lack of access to screening and psychiatric expertise contributes to undertreatment, but studies also found that mothers are ambivalent about the use of psychotropic medications during pregnancy or while breastfeeding (Kim et al. 2015; Myczkowski et al. 2012; Susser et al. 2016). Thus, modalities such as TMS may be important options, with advantages including the lack of systemic effects that could theoretically affect a developing fetus or a breastfeeding infant. Furthermore, no concurrent medications are administered with TMS, whereas electroconvulsive therapy (ECT) requires anesthetic agents (Kim et al. 2015; Myczkowski et al. 2012). The existing published literature that focuses on TMS for perinatal depression is summarized in Table 4–3.

Early results are promising and underscore the necessity for further systematic research. A single-center RCT showed efficacy for 1-Hz TMS applied to the right DLPFC for women with MDD during the second and third trimesters of pregnancy. Three women in the active group had late preterm births. Otherwise, infant outcomes did not differ significantly among the active and sham TMS groups (Kim et al. 2019).

In other case studies and open-label trials, a variety of low- and high-frequency dosing schedules, coil locations (left, right, and sequential bilateral DLPFC), and relatively brief treatment courses were undertaken in all trimesters, as well as postpartum. Initial results indicate good outcomes in terms of depressive symptom improvement and maternal-fetal health. Early experience indicates that after 24 weeks of pregnancy, women receiving TMS should be positioned on their left side with a wedge cushion under the right lower back for a 30° tilt to avoid inferior vena cava compression syndrome, thus mitigating supine hypotension (Kim and Wang 2014; Kim et al. 2015). Researchers examined children (mean age=32.4 months; range=16–64 months) of mothers who had received TMS for depression during pregnancy and a control group of children (mean age=29.04 months; range=14–63 months) whose mothers had a history of untreated depression during pregnancy. In the TMS-treated group, two infants had jaundice, and one infant had febrile convulsions. In the untreated group, three infants had jaundice, and one infant had low birth weight. Mothers who were treated with TMS reported a perceived language delay in their children, but there was no actual difference when they were compared with children of untreated mothers. Results suggested that no cognitive or motor delays were associated with prenatal TMS treatment for depression (Eryılmaz et al. 2015).

Within the limited body of research for TMS during pregnancy, no notable adverse effects on the fetus or pregnancy were identified. However, we found no publications addressing measurements of fetal stress (e.g., fetal heart rate) or uterine activity during TMS treatment. Although these

Table 4–3. Published experience with transcranial magnetic stimulation (TMS) for perinatal depression

Reference	N	Status of pregnancy	Treatment location	Frequency; intensity	Sessions	Outcomes
Kim et al. 2011	10	Second or third trimester	R-DLPFC	1 Hz; 100% MT	20	Seven patients responded (HDRS-17). No adverse maternal or fetal events occurred. Four patients had a mild headache.
Myczkowski et al. 2012	14	Postpartum	L-DLPFC	5 Hz; 120% MT or sham TMS	20	Active TMS yielded improvement at week 6 (HDRS-17). Two patients had mild scalp pain. No other side effects were reported.
Hızlı Sayar et al. 2014	30	First, second, and third trimesters	L-DLPFC	25 Hz; 100% MT	18	Mean HDRS-17 scores decreased significantly after treatment. One patient withdrew early. No adverse maternal or fetal events occurred.
Kim et al. 2019	22	Second or third trimester	R-DLPFC	1 Hz; 100% MT	20	HDRS-17 scores decreased significantly with active TMS compared with sham treatment.

Note. HDRS-17 and HDRS-24=Hamilton Depression Rating Scale, 17 items and 24 items, respectively; L-DLPFC=left dorsolateral prefrontal cortex; MT=motor threshold; R-DLPFC=right dorsolateral prefrontal cortex.

early results are encouraging (Eryılmaz et al. 2015; Kim et al. 2015), further comprehensive studies are necessary to explore the potential effects of TMS on pregnant patients and their fetuses to conclusively determine its safety and efficacy. Notably, we could not find any published reports of use of the deep TMS H-coil system in this population. Table 4–4 reviews clinical considerations for the use of TMS in treating perinatal depression.

Clinical Vignette 2

A 29-year-old woman in week 24 of pregnancy presented with severe symptoms of major depression, including low mood, amotivation, anhedonia, initial insomnia, low self-esteem, decreased appetite, and passive suicidal thoughts. Weekly CBT sessions for the past 2 months did not improve her symptoms. Her partner and family had concerns about her adherence to prenatal care and health maintenance. Even though she had a history of one previous major depressive episode with a good response to fluoxetine, she was not willing to initiate treatment with antidepressant medication during her pregnancy because of concerns about adverse events. At the obstetrician's recommendation, healthy lifestyle interventions and additional family support were instituted, and the patient consulted a psychiatrist with TMS experience. The psychiatrist reviewed the initial evidence for safety and effectiveness of TMS with the patient, her partner, and the patient's obstetrician. The TMS clinician recommended a 4-week course of daily 1-Hz treatments delivered over the right DLPFC. During each session, to avoid supine hypotension, the patient rested on a cushion under her right lower lumbar region for a 30° tilt toward her left side. The patient tolerated treatments with no adverse effects. Serial ratings with the Quick Inventory of Depressive Symptomatology—Self Report (QIDS-SR), as well as the patient's and her partner's reports, indicated improvement in depressive symptoms. The patient delivered a full-term, healthy female infant with no complications. At postnatal follow-up, the patient was euthymic, and both mother and infant were doing well.

Adolescent Depression

Adolescent MDD is a relatively common, heterogeneous, and undertreated disorder. Worldwide, it presents a significant public health problem and is a primary contributing factor to completed suicide, a leading cause of death in this age group. On an individual level, depressive episodes in adolescents also lead to considerable functional impairment, academic struggles, substance use, social dysfunction, teenage pregnancy, lifelong disease burden, and exposure to ineffective treatments. Evidence-based psychotherapeutic approaches such as CBT and SSRIs are considered first-line treatment approaches; however, up to 40% of youths may not respond to them. Treatment with CBT and SSRIs may also fail to address relevant neurodevelopmental pathophysiology. Among adolescents who do not

Table 4–4. Considerations for transcranial magnetic stimulation (TMS) treatment of perinatal depression

Perinatal depression is common, impairing, and treatable.

Suboptimal therapy produces substantial negative effects for mothers, developing fetuses, and infants.

Standard approaches are psychotherapy (e.g., cognitive-behavioral therapy or interpersonal therapy), selective serotonin reuptake inhibitors, or a combination of both.

Wellness strategies (exercise, stress management, bolstering family support, and assessing family health) are important aspects of treatment.

When possible, exposure to medications and untreated depressive episodes should be minimized.

Preliminary experience with TMS for both antepartum and postpartum depression is encouraging.

The initial evaluation for TMS should include input from family, an obstetrician, a primary psychiatrist, and a TMS expert.

The limits of the existing evidence base regarding TMS and the risks of untreated depression should be reviewed with patients and families to assist with an informed decision about treatment.

A variety of TMS dosing strategies were used with good results in terms of effectiveness, as well as maternal and fetal health.

Right-sided low-frequency TMS has the most evidence to date and might be the optimal approach.

Relatively brief treatment courses (15–20 sessions) may be effective.

Beyond 24 weeks of pregnancy, a 30° left tilt position while the patient is receiving TMS might mitigate supine hypotension.

Clinicians delivering TMS may need to use creative scheduling practices and resources to serve this population in the context of potential prenatal or childcare demands.

respond to an initial antidepressant trial, fewer than half will experience improvement with a second antidepressant treatment (Brent et al. 2008). These factors, along with ongoing controversies regarding the safety and effectiveness of antidepressants for MDD in adolescents, accentuate the need for alternative treatment options (Cipriani et al. 2016). Existing published studies of TMS for adolescent depression are reviewed in Table 4–5.

Recent systematic reviews and meta-analyses concluded that TMS may be effective and tolerable for treatment-resistant depression (TRD) in adolescents (Qiu et al. 2023). However, earlier enthusiasm was tempered by caution because of limited evidence and the shortcomings of available study data. Many initial studies consisted of case reports or unblinded, open-label trials with inadequate sample sizes. For example, the largest

Table 4–5. Published experience with transcranial magnetic stimulation for adolescent depression

Reference	N	Mean age (range)	Treatment location	Frequency; intensity	Pulses/session; stimulus train; number of trains	Sessions	Duration (weeks)	Outcomes
Wall et al. 2016	10	15.9 (13–17)	L-DLPFC	10 Hz; 120% MT	3,000 pulses; 40 stimulations; 75 trains	30	8	Improvement in mean depressive symptom severity with CDRS-R after 10, 20, and 30 treatments and at 6-month follow-up. Scalp discomfort, headaches, dizziness, musculoskeletal discomfort, eye twitching, and nausea reported, with 1 participant withdrawing during first session because of discomfort.
MacMaster et al. 2019	32	17.6 (13–21)	L-DLPFC	10 Hz; 120% MT	3,000 pulses; 40 stimulations; 75 trains	15	2	Improvement in mean depressive symptom severity with HDRS: 56% response, 44% remission. No serious adverse events: 19% mild to moderate headaches, 16% mild neck pain.

Table 4–5. Published experience with transcranial magnetic stimulation for adolescent depression *(continued)*

Reference	N	Mean age (range)	Treatment location	Frequency; intensity	Pulses/session; stimulus train; number of trains	Sessions	Duration (weeks)	Outcomes
Dhami et al. 2019	20	20.9 (16–24)	L-DLPFC (iTBS); R-DLPFC (cTBS)	Theta burst stimulation; 80% MT	1,800 pulses iTBS; 1,800 pulses cTBS	10	2	Significant reduction in depressive symptoms: 20% response, 10% remission. No safety or tolerability concerns.
Croarkin et al. 2021	103	Active: 17.6; sham: 17.1 (12–21)	L-DLPFC	10 Hz; 120% MT	3,000 pulses; 40 stimulations; 75 trains	30	6	No significant differences in efficacy, tolerability, or safety between active and sham treatment. Active: 41.7% response, 29.2% remission. Sham: 36.4% response, 29.0% remission.

Note. CDRS-R=Children's Depression Rating Scale—Revised; cTBS=continuous theta burst stimulation; HDRS=Hamilton Depression Rating Scale; iTBS=intermittent theta burst stimulation; L-DLPFC=left dorsolateral prefrontal cortex; MT=motor threshold; R-DLPFC=right dorsolateral prefrontal cortex.

RCT failed to find a significant difference in effectiveness between TMS and sham TMS for treating depression, with both groups showing improvements in depressive symptoms but no superiority for active TMS. This study, adapted from an adult protocol, was likely underpowered (Croarkin et al. 2021).

However, a new development has shifted the landscape: the FDA issued 510(k) premarket notification to Neuronetics on March 22, 2024, granting clearance for TMS in adolescents (U.S. Food and Drug Administration 2024). NeuroStar Advanced Therapy is now indicated as an adjunct for the treatment of MDD in adolescent patients ages 15–21. The clearance was based on real-world data submitted to the FDA by Neuronetics. In this dataset of 1,169 adolescents, 78% showed clinically meaningful improvements in depression severity. These comprehensive data, combined with clinical trial data, confirmed that TMS is effective and safe when used as an adjunct to antidepressant therapy in adolescents.

In general, dosing strategies parallel clinical practice for adults with depression. For example, various published protocols for treating adolescents offered up to 30 sessions of 10-Hz TMS at 80%–120% motor threshold applied over the left DLPFC. In most studies, TMS was an adjunct to psychotropic medications (Qiu et al. 2023). One effort used an MRI-guided approach for TMS coil localization, but the added clinical benefit of this approach is uncertain (Wall et al. 2016). One study examined sequential bilateral TBS dosing (MacMaster et al. 2019) because this approach may have advantages with respect to time burden for patients, safety, and clinical effects.

Although these results are encouraging for the application of TMS in adolescent TRD, many unanswered questions and challenges remain. Some adolescents and families might favor the use of TMS over medication, but the data to guide this approach are limited. Ideally, future studies of TMS in adolescents and clinical registry efforts will standardize approaches for comparison across sites. They should also focus on methods to better understand and reduce placebo response, precision dosing and targeting approaches, and treatment of more well-defined depressive phenotypes.

Published data on ECT in adolescents suggest that it is a safe and effective treatment for severe, treatment-resistant psychiatric disorders. Considerations in referring an adolescent for ECT include the presence of severe depression, bipolar disorder, or schizophrenia spectrum illnesses. In any of these disorders, symptoms should be persistent, severe, and life-threatening. Examples include failure to eat and take fluids, imminent suicidality, catatonia, and psychosis. Symptoms also should show resistance to at least two optimal trials of appropriate pharmacotherapy with evidence-based psychotherapeutic approaches. In most circumstances, adolescents receiving ECT are hospitalized. Notably, a variety of state and institutional guidelines restrict access to ECT for adolescents in some settings (Puffer et al. 2016).

In this context, more studies and experience with ECT and TMS for adolescent depression are needed. In the meantime, clinical factors, pragmatic considerations, and existing literature suggest that these two modalities are treatment options for distinct populations, depending on symptom severity and acuity.

With any off-label or investigational therapy, adolescents, families, and clinicians should temper enthusiasm with careful consideration of the risk-benefit ratio and the limits of existing evidence. Several commentaries focused on the promise and perils of brain stimulation approaches such as TMS during brain development (Davis 2014; Geddes 2015). The potential differences in myelination, neuroanatomy, and electrical field distributions in youths compared with adults present challenges in anticipating the broad effects of stimulation. Although initial systematic reviews suggested that TMS has a favorable side-effect profile in youths, longer-term data are lacking. A case report (Cullen et al. 2016) of an induced seizure with deep TMS also documented the need for future dose-finding research in adolescent depression (see Chapter 5, "Risk Management Issues in Transcranial Magnetic Stimulation for Treatment of Major Depression"). Although neurodevelopmentally informed and translational studies are currently lacking, TMS will likely offer an important treatment option for adolescent depression in the future. It is important, however, to consider that current, ubiquitous, off-label practices with polypharmacy are also poorly understood (Kearns and Hawley 2014) and, compared with TMS, could present a greater side-effect burden and increased risk for adolescents. Table 4–6 reviews key considerations for clinicians, patients, and families contemplating the use of TMS for depression in adolescents.

Clinical Vignette 3

A 17-year-old girl with a history of recurrent MDD and generalized anxiety disorder since age 11 years presented for treatment. Numerous trials of psychotherapy and adequate trials of psychotropic medications (e.g., fluoxetine, escitalopram, venlafaxine, desvenlafaxine, buspirone, lamotrigine, quetiapine, and aripiprazole) guided by prior pharmacogenomic testing were ineffective or poorly tolerated. At the time of consultation, she was taking sertraline (100 mg/day) and reported some relief in terms of her anxiety, but she was not comfortable increasing the dosage because

Table 4–6. Considerations for transcranial magnetic stimulation (TMS) treatment of adolescent depression

NeuroStar Advanced Therapy is now indicated as an adjunct for the treatment of major depressive disorder (MDD) in adolescent patients ages 15–21.

Psychotropic medications are also often prescribed off-label for children and adolescents.

Initial experience suggests that TMS may have a low side-effect burden in adolescents.

A 6-week period of left prefrontal TMS at 10 Hz in adolescents appears to be safe and tolerable.

Long-term safety studies of TMS in adolescents are lacking.

Baseline and follow-up assessment of symptom severity should include standardized rating scales.

A comprehensive treatment history should be obtained to evaluate prior interventions and adherence.

Comorbidity should be assessed and carefully considered.

Historical suicidal behavior should be characterized, and current suicidality should be evaluated.

Patients with *mild symptom severity* often respond to psychoeducation, supportive interventions, and adequate trials of evidence-based psychotherapies such as CBT and IPT.

Patients with *moderate to severe symptom severity* often respond to pharmacotherapy, evidence-based psychotherapies such as CBT and IPT, or their combination.

At a minimum, treatment resistance should be defined in the context of an adequate prior antidepressant trial (e.g., fluoxetine, 20–40 mg/day, for at least 8 weeks).

Suicidality should be assessed carefully during any treatment.

A meticulous informed consent process for adolescents and parents is imperative. It should impart understanding of the relevant limits of the evidence base for TMS in adolescents and the paucity of long-term safety data. Off-label practices with antidepressant medications and polypharmacy can be discussed in this context to compare evidence bases and potential tolerability.

Patient and parent preferences should be carefully considered.

Although emerging studies are examining TBS treatments for adolescents, extant published experience in adolescent depression primarily involves 10-Hz TMS applied over the left dorsolateral prefrontal cortex.

Previous studies of TMS in adolescent depression often applied TMS as an adjunctive treatment to pharmacotherapy in small samples of participants.